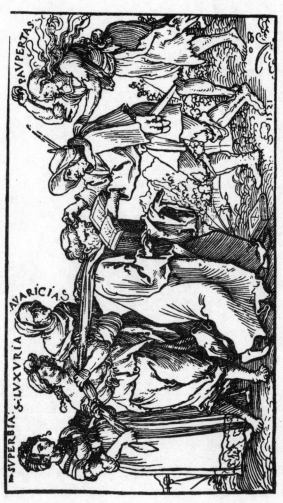

Frontispiece: Anticlerical German broadsheet from 1521 by Hans Sebald Beham, 'Allegory of Monastic Orders', showing a friar, representing the voluntary poor, being ruled by the vices of Pride (Superbia), Luxury (Luxuria) and Greed (Avaricia). The rightful, involuntary lay poor, in rags ('the image of Christ') is urged on by Poverty (Paupertas) to force the friar, who has wrongfully encroached on the charity for the poor, to literally eat the Word of the Bible.

Courtesy of Österreichische Nationalbibliothek, Vienna.

Health Care and Poor Relief in Protestant Europe 1500–1700

STUDIES IN THE SOCIAL HISTORY OF MEDICINE
Series Editors: Jonathan Barry and Bernard Harris

In recent years, the social history of medicine has become recognised as a major field of historical enquiry. Aspects of health, disease, and medical care now attract the attention not only of social historians but also of researchers in a broad spectrum of historical and social science disciplines. The Society for the Social History of Medicine, founded in 1969, is an interdisciplinary body, based in Great Britain but international in membership. It exists to forward a wide-ranging view of the history of medicine, concerned equally with biological aspects of normal life, experience of and attitudes of illness, medical thought and treatment, and systems of medical care. Although frequently bearing on current issues, this interpretation of the subject makes primary reference to historical context and contemporary priorities. The intention is not to promote a sub-specialism but to conduct research according to the standards and intelligibility required of history in general. The Society publishes a journal, *Social History of Medicine*, and holds at least three conferences a year. Its series, Studies in the Social History of Medicine, does not represent publication of its proceedings, but comprises volumes on selected themes, often arising out of conferences but subsequently developed by the editors.

Life, Death and the Elderly
Edited by Margaret Pelling and Richard M. Smith

Medicine and Charity Before the Welfare State
Edited by Jonathan Barry and Colin Jones

In the Name of the Child
Edited by Roger Cooter

Reassessing Foucault
Power, Medicine and the Body
Edited by Colin Jones and Roy Porter

From Idiocy to Mental Deficiency
Edited by David Wright and Anne Digby

Nutrition in Britain
Edited by David F. Smith

Health Care and Poor Relief in Protestant Europe 1500–1700

Edited by Ole Peter Grell and
Andrew Cunningham

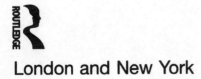

London and New York

First published 1997
by Routledge
11 New Fetter Lane, London EC4P 4EE

Simultaneously published in the USA and Canada
by Routledge
29 West 35th Street, New York, NY 10001

Typeset in Garamond by Routledge
Printed and bound in Great Britain by
Mackays of Chatham PLC, Chatham, Kent

British Library Cataloguing in Publication Data
A catalogue record for this book is available from the British Library

Library of Congress Cataloguing in Publication Data
A catalogue record for this book has been requested

ISBN 0–415–12130–2

Contents

List of contributors

Maria Bogucka Department of History, Polish Academy of Sciences, Warsaw, Poland

Andrew Cunningham Wellcome Unit for the History of Medicine, University of Cambridge

Ole Peter Grell Wellcome Unit for the History of Medicine, University of Cambridge

Jonathan I. Israel Department of History, University College, London

Robert Jütte Institut für Geschichte der Medizin der Robert Bosch Stiftung, University of Stuttgart, Germany

E. I. Kouri Department of History, University of Helsinki, Finland

E. Ladewig Petersen Department of History, University of Odense, Denmark

Rosalind Mitchison Department of History, University of Edinburgh

Thomas Riis Department of History, University of Kiel, Germany

Paul Slack Principal of Linacre College, Oxford

Hugo Soly Department of History, Free University of Brussels, Belgium

Preface

Most of the papers included in this volume were presented at a conference entitled *Health Care Provision and Poor Relief in the Baltic and North Sea Region 1500–1700*, held in Odense, Denmark, in September 1994. The conference was organised jointly by the Danish Committee for the History of Towns, which was then chaired by Professor Thomas Riis, Department of History, University of Kiel, Germany; and the Wellcome Unit for the History of Medicine at the University of Cambridge. We should like to thank the University of Odense for hosting this conference, and the participants who contributed to what proved a stimulating event.

In order to give this volume a fuller geographical and historical range, two papers which were not presented at the conference have been added, and the editors should like to thank those contributors who kindly offered to contribute to this volume at a later date.

We should also like to take this opportunity to thank the Wellcome Trust and Nordisk Kulturfond for generous financial support which made the conference possible.

Ole Peter Grell and Andrew Cunningham
Cambridge, May 1996

Chapter 1

The Reformation and changes in welfare provision in early modern Northern Europe

Ole Peter Grell and Andrew Cunningham

This volume intends to provide a comparative survey of the welfare provisions available to the poor and sick in early modern, Protestant Northern Europe. It also explores the relationship between Protestantism and reform on the one hand and the changes in health care provision, that is 'professional' medical care, nursing and hospitals, on the other. The volume draws attention to the fact that the major context of health care provision in the early modern period was poor relief, which in turn has to be seen within the context of the ideology of the Reformation.

Geographically it deals with the countries surrounding the North Sea and the Baltic. Such a choice is fully justified by the contemporary network of economic, religious, and political contacts which linked this region together. Furthermore, apart from Antwerp, which became a Calvinist centre only from the mid-1570s until 1585, it is also an area where the Protestant Reformation made a lasting impact. Obviously the eleven chapters presented here cannot deal exhaustively with health care provision and poor relief in all these countries, particularly since issues such as medical care have received only scant attention within most of the national historiographies covered here. However, in the case of England, which is unique in having seen the publication of a considerable number of works dealing with the country's social and medical history in the early modern period over the last three decades, the problem is the exact opposite: how to include it all.[1]

Seen exclusively within an Anglo-Saxon social-medical historiography, the chapters presented in this volume with their deliberate focus on urban and institutional welfare reforms in the early modern period, may present a contrast with more present-centred emphases on outdoor assistance, the poor themselves, and gender. However, the lack of detailed studies in most of the region with which this volume is concerned would have rendered such an approach dubious if not impossible. Thus in order to produce a truly comparative volume, an urban, institutional focus placed within the context of the Protestant Reformation offers the most promising parameters.

Without denying the significance of the serious social and economic changes which affected Western Europe in the sixteenth- and seventeenth centuries, most of the contributors to this volume have serious reservations about the traditional or conventional association between economic change and welfare reforms.[2] Apart from major social eruptions, in the form of rebellions, it is far from clear whether it was economic boom or slump which stimulated reforms. Instead a majority of the chapters in this volume emphasise the role and importance of ideology and politics and undoubtedly support the call for a revised and a renewed emphasis on the significance of the Protestant Reformation for the speed and thoroughness of the reforms in health care and poor relief in early modern Northern Europe as expressed in Chapter 2 of this volume.

That poverty and disease represented two sides of the same coin is well known, but that medical treatment and care formed an important part of poor relief and charity well before the so-called medicalisation of the eighteenth century has yet to be fully appreciated. Furthermore, medical treatment and care was not restricted to inmates of poor houses and hospitals, but was available to those supported at home – the house poor – as Robert Jütte shows in the case of the cities of Hamburg, Lübeck and Bremen.[3] The medical care available to the poor in the cities of Northern Germany would appear to have been similar to that on offer to the poor in the wealthy London parish of St Bartholomew's Exchange in the late sixteenth- and seventeenth centuries.[4] It was a two-track system of health care. One, the most basic, was run by the poor themselves. They provided a nursing service for those of their fellow-pensioners who fell ill or were injured, paid for by the parish. This was a system which appears to have been mutually beneficial to both the poor and the parish, as in the case of the widow Hasard who received several payments of one pound during the autumn of 1640 for looking after a poor man who had broken his leg. While supporting its poor the parish was able to provide health care for its sick and invalid.

The other track consisted of 'professional' medicine, seeking out and paying for the advice and drugs provided by physicians, surgeons and apothecaries. The financial help given to poor parishioners who sought 'professional' medical help was, as was the case in Hamburg and Bremen, not given automatically or by right, but had to be petitioned for. In many instances the poor would have had to find the necessary money themselves in the first instance only to be reimbursed by the parish or the overseers at a later date. Even so, it is noteworthy that the poor were not automatically excluded from 'professional' medical care despite the fact that it was generally considered costly.

Even if Protestantism and the Reformation cannot lay sole claim to having caused the reforms of poor relief and health care which occured in the sixteenth- and seventeenth centuries in Protestant Western Europe, the speed and thoroughness with which they were undertaken would not have been imaginable without the theological rationale which the Protestant reformers gave to these reforms.[5] As argued by Ole Peter Grell, it is time for a revision of the 1960s historiography, which tended to see the welfare reforms as being solely humanist and civic in origin and used an interpretation based on an often simplistic economic and social determinism.[6]

Begging had been at the centre of the medieval practice of charity, not least because of the teachings of Francis of Asissi and other Franciscans such as Bernardino of Siena who had emphasised that begging most fully expressed a person's relationship with God. However, by the end of the fifteenth century the humility traditionally associated with the poor begging for alms was rapidly disappearing, not least because of their numerical increase. Instead begging became increasingly associated with the aggression and threat represented by sturdy beggars and vagrants. Furthermore the motives and humility of the mendicant orders, the leading representatives of the voluntary poor, were increasingly questioned by the urban laity. That the mendicant orders and their begging became a main target for Luther and the other reformers with their emphasis on faith and grace cannot surprise. The begging of these voluntary poor was considered presumptuous and blasphemous, apart from providing unfair competition to the truly needy. Poverty was for God to designate, not to be chosen as a particularly blessed state by friars and priests. It is undoubtedly in this confrontation with and rejection of voluntary, ecclesiastical poverty, based on a theology of faith and grace, that the Protestant ambition and need to develop a clear distinction between the deserving and undeserving poor is rooted. According to Protestants, voluntary or perceived voluntary poverty, whether lay or ecclesiastical, made a mockery of real poverty, which fell to the Christian commonwealth to tackle as an expression of neighbourly love, but not in order to earn points towards one's salvation, towards which humanity by definition was unable to contribute. Consequently, Protestants strove to eliminate all begging rather than just trying to regulate and control it, which tended to be the Catholic solution.

Not surprisingly Catholic contemporaries accused Protestant communities of trying drastically to limit the numbers of deserving poor. In the main they were probably correct in their perception of Protestant communities seeking to restrict their charity to the residential, authentic and morally upright poor.[7] Plenty of examples can be found of Protestant communities refusing to assist the sick and needy for moral reasons. In Delft in the United Provinces the poor assisted by the Reformed Church were not allowed to frequent inns, while in 1622 the consistory of the church in Alkmaar refused to pay for the medical treatment of a poor woman whose immoral living had caused her to be infected with the pox.[8] However, this is far from the whole picture. Occasionally, the sense of *caritas* might override the urge to impose social discipline, and assistance would be offered despite serious moral shortcomings. In August 1579 a certain Magdelene Vondelings appeared before the consistory of the Dutch Reformed Church in London. She had been excommunicated and now wanted to be reconciled with the community and re-admitted to the communion table. The consistory rejected her request, pointing out that she had fallen pregnant as a result of an illicit affair with a young man. However, they listened sympathetically to her complaints of ill health and homelessness, and having consoled her with 'words from the Bible' they recommended her case to the deacons for assistance.[9]

THE SIGNIFICANCE OF REFORMED EMIGRATION AND RE-EMIGRATION FOR THE CHANGES IN WELFARE PROVISION IN THE UNITED PROVINCES AND IN ANTWERP

The religious and social significance of Reformed emigration from the Southern Netherlands and the period of re-emigration that followed (and which eventually saw many of those who had sought refuge in England and Germany return to the Netherlands) can hardly be overstated with regard to the changes in health care and poor relief which took place in Northern Europe from the second half of the sixteenth century onwards. The wealth of material and documentation relating to the Dutch exile community in London provides us with a particularly valuable example of how these communities functioned. The caring approach of the first generation of ministers and elders in the Dutch Reformed community in London even towards those of their poor who caused offence and difficulties was often remarkable. Faced in December 1573 with a woman who had insulted the deacons and expressed her dissatisfaction with the relief offered to her and her four children – five shillings a month – while publicly stating that she had no intent of taking her complaints either to the church or the consistory, because, according to her, poor people could expect no justice or fair treatment there, the consistory members, instead of severely disciplining her, dealt patiently with her, eventually reconciling her with the deacons and the community.[10]

The poor belonging to the Dutch Reformed communities were, like their Lutheran counterparts, expected to refrain from begging in return for the relief provided by their community. A further aspect of the 'discipline' they had to accept in order to receive alms was the obligation to open their homes to regular visits and inspections by the deacons, plus their obligation to keep the deacons informed about their financial situation. However, these regular home visits by the deacons did not only serve to impose social discipline and prevent abuse. In many communities they also provided an occasion for the deacons to hand out their charity in a non-public and discreet manner. This was an approach which served to minimise the stigma attached to poor relief and which made sure that assistance also reached the honourable poor who might feel ashamed to come forward in public. Thus in June 1572, the minister to the Dutch Church in London, Jooris Wybo, suggested to the consistory that in future alms should be distributed to the poor in their homes and not in the church. He also suggested that the regular house visits paid to all members by one of the ministers accompanied by the local elder should in future include a deacon, in order to make sure that the honourable poor who were hesitant to come forward could be included in the community's charity.[11] It was obviously important for the poor to try and hang on to what little honour they had left. The totally destitute often did their utmost to avoid the stigma attached to moving into the poorhouse even if this institution could provide them with a guarantee of shelter and food. Many of the poor were happy to receive outdoor relief while the prospect of the poorhouse clearly represented a further drop in social prestige and freedom from which the poor saw little chance of recovering. Thus in 1633 the deacons of Austin Friars in London had to request the assistance of the elders and ministers in forcing some of the community's poor to move into the poorhouse.[12]

After 1572, when the Dutch Revolt had become essentially a Protestant revolt, and the Reformed Church was actively establishing itself within the United Provinces, two avenues of relief were open to the poor in the rebellious north apart from begging. They could approach the lay overseers of the poor who were employed by the local magistracies, who had taken over the houses of the Holy Spirit and with them the patrimony of the Catholic Church. Or they could try their luck with the newly appointed deacons in most urban communities who collected money for the poor immediately after the services and conducted door-to-door collections among members and sympathisers of the Reformed faith, which were not exclusively intended for members.

In reality, however, it is difficult to draw a distinction between lay and Reformed charity in the United Provinces. In some places such as Leiden and Enkhuizen all income from former Catholic charities and religious establishments and from gifts and collections were gathered in a common chest which was administered jointly by the overseers and the deacons, but with the civil authorities dominating. Since faith did not enter into the question of whether or not someone qualified for relief, such a regime might occasionally cause unexpected problems. Thus godly, Reformed refugees from the Southern Netherlands might find themselves excluded from receiving relief, because they failed to fulfill the important criteria of residence in order to be included among the deserving poor. In particular this seems to have occurred in villages with a Catholic majority and resulted in complaints about the overseers favouring 'those of the Popish religion'.[13] The deacons' account book for the community of Hazerswoude near Leiden covering the years 1620–5 may well offer a guide to how the money collected for the poor and sick was spent by the Reformed communities in the Dutch Republic. Poor relief was generally offered on a continuous or longer-term basis whereas one-off assistance tended to be given to the sick and to women who had recently given birth.

Even in cities such as Amsterdam where the lay overseers and deacons operated totally separately and where the deacons were expected to care for members of their congregations while the city officials dealt with other residents of the city, the magistracy kept a controlling hand on the till. The city council remained well represented within the consistory during most of the late sixteenth- and seventeenth century, a fair number of councillors served regularly as elders and deacons, while a percentage of church collections were always handed over to the lay overseers of the poor. The deacons in major Dutch cities such as Haarlem and Amsterdam seem to have been able to dispose of large amounts of money for charitable purposes during this period. In Amsterdam the Reformed community was able to distribute 10,000 guilders in 1587, 70,000 guilders in 1608, 140,000 guilders in 1625 and 250,000 guilders in 1645 to the poor and sick.[14] Despite their primary concern for the welfare of members the deacons never excluded other needy. Travellers with attestations, proving their membership of Reformed communities in other towns and cities, were assisted as were many travellers without such papers, especially soldiers who had served in the war against the Spaniards.

The wealth and ability to provide poor relief of the Reformed Church in Amsterdam, combined with the explosive growth of the city from the late 1580s onwards, caused problems for the deacons. Amsterdam was attracting a continuous stream of immigrants and migrants who were looking for opportunities and employment in the city and who, if they possessed valid attestations from other Reformed communities, could lay some claim to poor relief from the church. Many fell on hard times and must have placed an increasing burden on the community's resources. In order to protect itself and avoid becoming an easy touch for the poor from other Reformed communities looking for employment in the city, the Amsterdam church decided in 1599 that new members had to serve a trial membership of two to three months before they qualified for poor relief from the church.[15]

This problem was far from unique to the Reformed community of Amsterdam in this period. The Dutch Reformed community in London found itself in a similar situation in the 1630s. Here as in Amsterdam the problem was rooted in the city's rapid growth, attracting large numbers of new migrants looking for work, combined with the Dutch community's renowned system of poor relief. For the many poor and destitute seeking employment this offered an opportunity they could not afford to miss. A membership of the Dutch Church in Austin Friars might provide them with an insurance against poverty and disease. In December 1635 a consistory meeting decided to assess and carefully evaluate new membership applications in order to avoid accepting people who might become a burden and who were seen as applying for membership solely to be able 'to live off the congregation'. At one point the meeting appears to have considered excluding new members who could provide no financial guarantees from receiving any assistance from the church within the first three years of their membership. This hardline approach, however, was eventually abandoned, but the meeting emphasised that under no circumstances were people 'who had shielded under the English' and taken communion in their local parish churches to be accepted as members, 'when they had reached old age and fallen on hard times'. Those, at least, who had failed the test of faith and left the community for the Anglican Church as a consequence of the pressure brought to bear on the foreign Reformed communities in England by Archbishop William Laud's campaign for uniformity were not to be rewarded for their cowardice and lack of religious backbone.[16]

As pointed out by Jonathan Israel, Dutch cultural and social influence in Northern Europe in the seventeenth century was in no small measure linked to the significant emigration of Protestant refugees from the Southern Netherlands who settled in England, Germany and Scandinavia in the years following the intervention of the Duke of Alva in 1567.[17] In England the Dutch and Walloon communities established in London in 1550 may well have provided inspiration for the hospital reforms initiated under Edward VI (as argued by Paul Slack), which saw five London hospitals restored or founded and the creation of the first European workhouse in the old royal palace of Bridewell in the 1550s.[18]

The Dutch and Walloon churches in London both maintained a poorhouse, which, at least in the case of the Dutch, was under the supervision of one of their deacons and was able to house around sixteen inmates.[19] But the bulk of the charity offered by the foreign Reformed churches came in the form of outdoor relief. Members supported by the foreign communities were expected to refrain from begging and to be regularly visited by the deacons not only to ensure that they were deserving in both a material and moral sense, but also to make sure that they received the assistance they needed and were entitled to. By the beginning of the seventeenth century the welfare provisions of the stranger churches in London had become not only a model for English Puritans, but were widely admired by those within the Church of England who had little sympathy for Calvinism. Thus Bishop Lancelot Andrews noted that the foreign Reformed communities in London were able 'to do so much good as not one of their poor is seen to ask in the streets', adding his regrets that 'this city, the harbourer and maintainer of them should not be able to do the same good'.[20]

Poor members of the Dutch community in London who fell ill could also expect to receive medical care paid for by the church. The leaders of the community appear to have been especially aware of the need to make sure that the services of surgeons and physicians were available when epidemics broke out. When a serious outbreak of plague took place in 1563, the Dutch Church in Austin Friars, which then had around 1,600 members spread across the city, decided to employ a physician-cum-surgeon, a certain Rembarts from Osnabrück, to look after the poor infected members of the community in particular. He was given a lump sum of sixteen shillings, four more than he had demanded, and promised a weekly salary of five shillings for looking after the poor, while the richer members were expected to pay for his services. Having failed to obtain the services of Mr Francoys, a surgeon who had fled from Hondschote in Flanders and settled in Sandwich, because the church had been hesitant in offering him a guaranteed salary, the leaders of the church evidently felt the need three days later to secure the services of Rembarts and another surgeon who promised to assist him if need arose. A couple of weeks later, in mid-July, the epidemic had accelerated so much that the consistory felt the need to recommend the services of Francoys to the community as a supplement to Rembarts and his assistant.

Furthermore poorer members were paid to serve as nurses and watchers while the church took the lead among all the Dutch Reformed churches by appointing two members as visitors of the sick, who were to assist the ministers in attending them. As opposed to the deacons, who were instructed to initiate weekly door-to-door collections in order to generate enough funds to pay for the relief and medical care provided and to pay particular attention to the growing needs of widows, orphans and the poor in the present crisis, the visitors of the sick, who were paid servants of the congregation, were charged with appointing nurses and watchers and instructed to help the sick in drawing up their wills and to offer them consolation and admonition.[21] They were, in other words, expected to cover both the spiritual and medical domains, hiring nurses and calling in the surgeon to attend the sick poor; but a clear emphasis was placed on the pastoral aspect of their duties. They evidently represent an interesting and early example of community medicine, and their role may well have become increasingly medical during epidemics in the seventeenth century, as the example of Rotterdam seems to indicate.[22]

The position as visitor of the sick was initially only intended to be filled in times of epidemics, not only in Austin Friars in London, but also in other towns and cities in the United Provinces such as Amsterdam, Leiden and Rotterdam, where this position was introduced in the 1580s and 90s. However, in London at least, it seems to have become semi-permanent around 1570, when Arnoldus de Stuer served the community, possibly as a consequence of the many epidemics affecting the City during this period. Plague had by then reappeared in the City, even if a serious epidemic did not result. The moral standing of the visitor was obviously important considering his responsibilities, as was that of the surgeon since both attended sick and dying members of the community. Thus rumours in 1563 that the surgeon appointed by the Walloon-French Church in London attended the sick in the company of a whore, convinced the consistory in Austin Friars not to recommend this man to their members.

Similarly, when in April 1570 De Stuer, together with the London community's surgeon Cornelis van der Maze, was found to have taken part in a drunken party in a plague-infected house in the Minories where the family received alms from the church, the consistory took immediate action. Rumours of this drinking bout, which had also involved the nurse Beatrice, who was not a member of the church but known to like a glass or two, and another two English women, were also rife among the English, to the detriment of the Dutch Church's standing in the City. Despite not being a member Beatrice was admonished, as were the surgeon and De Stuer. For De Stuer, who as visitor of the sick had been the person in authority at this gathering, the incident proved extremely damaging and probably lost him his job. His situation was not helped by the fact that some members had complained to the consistory about the visitor of the sick having taken over the ministers' traditional role of consoling the sick. This had proved particularly objectionable because the visitor's salary was paid out of the funds collected for the poor. De Stuer was consequently laid off and lots were drawn among the three ministers in order to find his replacement. As opposed to the public hostility to Reformed ministers visiting the plague-stricken in the United Provinces, which appears to have been instrumental in creating the position of visitor of the sick there, a significant number of members of the London Dutch community evidently preferred their ministers to fulfil this traditional role and visit the sick during epidemics, rather than see that responsibility passed on to a paid, lower official. However, the leadership of Austin Friars quickly decided to return to the system introduced in 1563 and new visitors of the sick were appointed. In terms of financing the salaries of these men a compromise was found. No longer were their salaries to be paid solely by the deacons. From now on the deacons would only provide half the visitors' salary while the other half was to be paid from funds held by the elders. In 1563 the two visitors had been paid ten shillings each per week by the elders while their successors in 1570 received twelve shillings per week paid joinly by elders and deacons.[23]

In London the position of visitor of the sick had become permanent by the early seventeenth century, having by then been amalgamated with the position of *voorleser* (reader) with an annual salary of twelve pounds. This pattern appears to have been followed in most of the United Provinces, especially in Zeeland and Holland, a few decades later. However, when plague struck London again in 1625 the Dutch Church refused to put the life of their regular visitor at risk and hired a temporary visitor of the plague-stricken. Thus by the early seventeenth century when the visitors of the sick had become permanent features within some Reformed communities, they may well have given rise to a similar institutional proliferation generated by the fear of plague which had originally led to the creation of their own positions in the first place.[24]

Protestant immigrants from the Southern Netherlands in particular were undoubtedly a major inspiration for reforms of poor relief and health care in the areas of North-Western Europe where they settled. But the exiled Reformed communities they formed in their exodus proved of similar if not greater magnitude when large numbers of these refugees returned to the Northern, as well as the Southern Netherlands in the 1570s. In the rebellious United Provinces their impact on reforms of poor relief and health care was paramount even if the lay magistracies retained financial control over such affairs in several cities.[25] The centralisation of

funds and resources, the appointment of committed lay administrators – deacons – and the arrangement of some sort of medical
provision for the poor and sick would have been difficult to imagine
in the Netherlands without the Reformed Church having obtained
the position of official church as a consequence of its leading role in
the Dutch Revolt.

Thus it is worth bearing in mind that Dr Nicolaes Tulp,
immortalised in Rembrandt's famous painting of him demonstrating his skill in anatomy, not only inspired the creation of the
Amsterdam *Collegium Medicum* in 1636, but served as an elder to the
Dutch Reformed Church in Amsterdam. Tulp, who had been a
member of the city council since 1622, became an elder in 1633.
The Amsterdam deacons were quick in drawing on his medical
expertise. During the seventeenth century a number of physicians,
surgeons and apothecaries regularly provided medical assistance to
the poor of the Amsterdam community on the request of the
deacons. They generally provided their services free of charge within
pre-determined areas of the city.

In 1633 the physician Françooys de Vick informed the deacons
that he was unable to continue to visit the sick poor in their
homes, which he had so far done for free, but that he was willing to
help those who wanted to consult him at his own house. In this
situation the deacons evidently felt the need to reorganise the
health care they provided for the poor of the community. Together
with Dr Tulp, who in his capacity of elder had been delegated to
assist them in these matters, the deacons decided to employ three
physicians, Johannes Grol, Dr Teulinck and Jacob Viverius. They
were each to be assisted by a surgeon and an apothecary while
serving the community. That Jacob Viverius, a Reformed refugee
from Ghent in the Southern Netherlands, should have offered his
services to the community, is not surprising. Viverius's strong
commitment to neighbourly love and Christian charity is in
evidence in his work on the plague first published in 1601, *De
Handt Godes of een Christelick verhael vande peste of Gaeve Godes*. In
1641 the Amsterdam church expanded this service to include a
fourth physician, presumably also assisted by a surgeon and an
apothecary. Apart from their Christian, Reformed commitment
these medical men may well also have been motivated by more
mundane reasons. Even if their services were offered for free, the
publicity they gained probably generated significant custom from
richer members who could pay for their services. Furthermore their

services did not go totally unremunerated by the church since the deacons awarded each of them a gift of a silver coin or medal to the value of fifty-eight guilders.[26]

The constant emigration and re-emigration of Reformed refugees from the southern Netherlands in particular, did not influence social policies and initiatives in Germany, Scandinavia and England exclusively, but also affected developments in the rebellious United Provinces. Thus when the city of Groningen finally joined the Union of Utrecht in 1594 and became part of the anti-Spanish front, it quickly resulted in a restructuring of the city's system of poor relief and health care provision. Apart from installing the Reformed Church as the only official church in the city and purging the city council of all its Catholic members, Groningen joining the Union of Utrecht caused a number of leading members of the Reformed community in Emden who had spent decades in exile to return.[27] Emden together with London had been the major centre for Dutch Reformed Protestantism in the years of exile between 1550 and the mid-1570s, and the return of these Calvinist exiles resulted in a transformation of the system of welfare in Groningen along Reformed lines. Deacons were elected, who were instructed to weed out the undeserving poor and make sure that the alms reached *den rechten Godes armen*. Undoubtedly several of the deacons appointed would have had previous experience from serving in the *Fremdendiaconie* in Emden.[28] The tasks of the Groningen deacons were identical to those of their colleagues in Emden and London. Detailed administrative regulations were laid down for their activities similar to those in London. They were to conduct collections at the church door after the services, plus door-to-door collections in their local areas. A register of income and expenditure was to be kept by the presiding deacon – the archdeacon. They were also to pay weekly visits to the poor who received alms, to assure themselves of their need and to review the continued assistance of all recipients of alms every six months. In what may well have been an arrangement particular to Groningen the deacons also received funds and loans from the city's eighteen guilds.

As in so many other Dutch cities the magistracy of Groningen continued to run its own system of poor relief in tandem with the new Calvinist system. Even for the magistracy, however, the Reformed takeover proved significant. Leading citizens had long been debating plans for establishing an orphanage, which had originally been drawn up in 1565, but nothing happened until five years after the city had joined the Union of Utrecht, when in 1599 the orphanage was finally established in the former Clarissa convent. Ten years later a workhouse was established, undoubtedly inspired by the Amsterdam equivalent which had been instituted in 1596. Finally in 1610 Groningen received its first Poor Order. All this was closely connected with the Calvinist Reformation which had been instituted in the city in 1594. Welfare reforms had evidently become a top priority for the new urban elite, who appear to have received much of their inspiration from former Emden exiles such as Doede van Amsweer, who had published his programme for a reform of charity, *Chritlijk Bedenckent unde dispotion van Armen Ordenung* in 1600. Using the metaphors of Luther and Zwingli for the lay, involuntary poor, as being the 'living images of God' van Amsweer instructed his readers to redirect their charity away from the Catholic altars and saints and instead to offer their gifts 'on the altar of the living' by putting their money in the poor box after having attended service.[29]

Due to the initial shortage of Reformed ministers the Groningen magistracy took the unusual step of appointing a visitor of the sick in 1599. His office, however, was discontinued by the time a sufficient number of ministers had been appointed to serve the community.

Surprisingly enough the hospitals in Groningen in their post-Reformation form continued to cater nearly exclusively for the elderly. Sick people were not admitted and only during the years of intensified warfare were sick and wounded soldiers exceptionally treated in these institutions. In times of epidemics a few plague victims could be treated in the small St Anthony's hospital. Instead, the city relied on a decentralised form of health care provision provided by the surgeons' guild which had come into existence in connection with the city's official Reformation in 1594. In 1601 the city fathers were seriously alarmed at the expenses incurred by the treatment of one of the children in the burghers' orphanage (an additional orphanage financed by the Reformed Church, but jointly supervised by church and magistracy, was to be established in 1621) and the magistracy made sure that the surgeons would in future offer their services for free in return for the privileges they enjoyed. From then on they were only to be reimbursed for the expenses they incurred on materials and drugs, while being excused from providing this free service for the sick poor in times of plague. But by 1631 the magistracy obviously felt a need to put its health care provision on a more institutional footing and consequently salaried surgeons were appointed to provide medical care in the city's two orphanages.[30]

A similar influence on social policy and welfare initiatives exerted by returning Reformed refugees can be detected in what Hugo Soly terms the Calvinist period in Antwerp.[31] By the mid-1570s the failure of the Spanish efforts to reconquer the Netherlands had become clear, Reformed confidence was growing and underground Reformed communities – 'the churches under the cross' – were established in places like Antwerp. When in 1576 the Pacification of Ghent brought a temporary halt to the hostilities and the persecution, a massive return of Calvinist refugees from London and Emden in particular resulted.[32] In 1582 the Dutch Reformed community in London provided the Antwerp church with one of its young ministers, Assuerus Regemorter, whose education the London church had sponsored. Like so many of his fellow refugees in London, Assuerus originated from Antwerp and when asked by the London consistory if he would accept the call from the Antwerp church he immediately accepted. Regemorter felt he had an obligation to help further the true faith in 'his father's city' where he himself had 'seen the truth and served as an elder for a period'.[33] In Antwerp he would have joined other Reformed exiles within the leadership of the church who had played a prominent role in the affairs of the London Dutch community, such as the wealthy merchant and scholar Johan Radermacher.

These returning Reformed exiles, more often than not with extensive direct experience of a smoothly running welfare machinery from service with their respective refugee churches abroad, brought important expertise back to Antwerp. The impact of their return combined with the Calvinist takeover may well help explain the 50 per cent increase in donations to the common chest at a time when the population in Antwerp declined by around 20 per cent. The new Calvinist management continued the already existing system of poor relief in Antwerp, but with some important differences. The Catholic religious orders were forbidden to collect and distribute alms and their funds were handed over to the common chest. A laicisation took place – the nuns running the St Elisabeth hospital were released from their vows and forced to wear secular clothes – merchants and master craftsmen took over the responsibility for the collection and distribution of all poor relief which was centralised in a common chest. Two surgeons were employed by the magistracy to look after the sick poor and a system of nursing created. Considering the considerable interest in medicine and health care demonstrated by Reformed leaders such as Johan Radermacher, whose extensive library contained a vast collection of medical works, this seems a natural development.[34] The surrender of Antwerp to Spanish forces in 1585, however, meant that the plans for a large new hospital and plague houses were never initiated.

Hugo Soly is undoubtedly right when pointing to the economic motives behind the Calvinist reforms of the boys' orphanage in Antwerp. But the ambition to apprentice as many orphans as possible to merchants and master craftsmen also had a strong religious imperative: namely to turn these boys into good Christian citizens who could serve and contribute to the Christian commonwealth in Antwerp.

Following the mass exodus of Reformed merchants and craftsmen from Antwerp in 1585, new initiatives within the field of poor relief and health care rested partly with new Counter-Reformation orders such as the Jesuits and partly with the magistracy, with clerical influence being gradually extended throughout the seventeenth century. Some Protestant initiatives were copied, such as the Amsterdam house of correction, and in 1613 Antwerp acquired a similar institution.

By the seventeenth century central government in the Spanish Netherlands, often on the instigation of the Archdukes, tried, not always succesfully, to reform and improve the welfare system. Thus a proposal by Archduke Albert in the late seventeenth century to introduce a poor tax or rate met with a negative response, while earlier suggestions by his predecessors for the creation of cheap public loan offices for the poor, so-called *Bergen van Barmhartigheid* to replace private pawnshops, were more successful. Modelled on the *Monti di Pieta* instituted in Italy in the fifteenth century, they were set up in fifteen cities in the the Spanish Netherlands in the early seventeenth century, even if the interest rates which they charged their customers – between 12 and 15 per cent – appear to have been well beyond the reach of the poorer sections of society.[35]

THE HANSEATIC CITIES OF NORTHERN GERMANY

In Hamburg, Bremen, and Lübeck, the Hanseatic towns of Northern Germany, medical care quickly became a significant part of the general welfare provision in the post-Reformation era.

Gradually, as Robert Jütte emphasises, medical care in these cities came to be seen as significant in preventing families from sinking into total impoverishment. Thus free medical care for the poor became a significant part of poor relief in these three cities well before the so-called medicalisation of the eighteenth century.[36]

This concern for the sick and invalid played a prominent part in Johannes Bugenhagen's Protestant church orders for Hamburg (1528) and Lübeck (1531). In the Hamburg Order they appeared in second place immediately after the honourable house poor who through no fault of their own found themselves in difficulties, as being those most deserving of assistance. Strangers and travellers, who were not otherwise entitled to support from the common chest, were to receive support in kind as well as in cash if they fell ill. The deacons in the four Hamburg parishes who had been elected the year prior to the introduction of the new Church Order were not only in charge of the outdoor relief in the city, but also of most of the indoor relief provided in the hospital of the Holy Spirit, Saint Ileseben Hospital and the smallpox hospital, the only exception being Saint George's Hospital which remained under the control of the magistracy. Furthermore, a large central hospital was to be created which should cater primarily for the poor and have a special separate section which could house plague victims.[37] Gradually, however, the deacons in Hamburg appear to have lost control over indoor relief, which instead came to rest with the magistracy.[38]

Similarly in Lübeck in 1531 Bugenhagen emphasised the obligation of the five senior deacons who presided over the distribution of alms from the common chest not only to focus their charity on the registered and known poor, but also to assist those who had suddenly fallen ill or poor women who had just given birth.[39] Likewise, it fell to the five senior deacons to establish a plague hospital inside the smallpox hospital, where total isolation of poor plague victims could be achieved. The senior deacons were obliged to provide such inmates with free nursing, food, firewood for heating, and bandages and clean bedding. One of the former monasteries in the city was to be converted into a joint poor house and hospital for those who had caught the pox. The deacons should finance these inmates' care and board if they themselves were destitute or without family and friends who were able and willing to contribute.[40] In case of a shortfall in the common chest in Lübeck Bugenhagen appears to have wanted to give the senior deacons the power to introduce some form of poor rate or tax on the wealthier citizens in order to raise the necessary funds.[41]

The Lutheran Church Order which was introduced in Bremen in 1534 made similar provisions to those in Hamburg and Lübeck. In cases where medical assistance was needed the Bremen Order did not discriminate between the resident poor and travellers. They were all entitled to help and could draw on the advice of physicians and surgeons paid for by the community, if their petition had been positively received by the deacons. The similarities in this respect between these Northern German Hanseatic cities and the cities in the United Provinces are evident and their rationale may well have been the same. This was a form of extended Christian charity which these communities could afford, since expenses towards medical care were more often than not short-term or one-off expenses.

That some of the health care initiatives taken in Bremen look remarkably similar to undertakings in the United Provinces should not surprise us. From the 1540s the Reformation in Bremen had developed in a distinctly Reformed direction, eventually leading to an open split between Lutherans and Reformed in 1561. In a situation where the Lutherans in Bremen wanted to introduce a new poor relief scheme, the Reformed party decided to seek the advice and assistance of the Marburg professor of theology Andreas Hyperius, who consequently produced his *De publica in pauperes beneficentia*, published posthumously in Basle in 1570, and translated into English two years later. Born in Ypres in Flanders in 1511 and educated at the local Latin school, whose headmaster had been instrumental in having the city's new poor relief order accepted in 1525, Hyperius is an excellent example of the futility of trying to separate humanist and Protestant influences and motives behind social reforms in the early phases of the Reformation. He was undoubtedly influenced by humanists such as Erasmus and Juan Luis Vives, but his thinking and theology were also strongly affected by leading reformers such as Martin Bucer and Johann Sturm. That Andreas Hyperius spent the years between 1537 and 1541 in England, in Oxford and Cambridge, may well explain why his tract was later translated into English. On his return to Germany Hyperius settled in Marburg where he became professor of theology in 1542 and remained until his death in 1564.

The main inspiration behind Hyperius's poor relief tract written on the request of the Reformed citizens of Bremen appears to have been the poor relief order introduced in his native Ypres in 1525.[42]

Hyperius wanted the responsibility for poor relief to be shared jointly between the magistracy and the Protestant/Reformed Church. Church leaders and civic leaders were to appoint three or four responsible people as overseers of the poor. These overseers were to visit the poor who received alms on a regular basis to assure themselves of their need and whether or not they needed further assistance such as medical care. They could in fact, funds permitting, pay visits to the sick poor in the company of the town physician to make sure that proper medical care was provided.[43] These aspects of Hyperius's proposal come remarkably close to the model followed in many towns and cities in the Dutch Republic a generation later.

In 1634 the deacons in Bremen attempted to get the resident physicians and surgeons to offer their services to the poor for free on a monthly rotational basis. This was a system which, as we have already seen, looks remarkably similar to that introduced in Groningen where the surgeons' guild performed a similar duty. Robert Jütte is undoubtedly correct when he emphasises the growing importance of medical care as a constitutive element of poor relief in the urban centres of early modern Germany.[44]

DENMARK

That the first clear distinction between the deserving and undeserving poor in Denmark should have appeared in the comprehensive legislation which King Christian II sought to introduce into his realm in 1522, only a year prior to his deposition and exile, is further proof of the influence of humanism and evangelical thinking on this monarch and his government. Thomas Riis, while emphasising the medieval antecedents for many of the changes in welfare provision which took place in Denmark in the sixteenth century, may well take a very bleak view of the lack of success on the ground of the reforms introduced in the wake of the Lutheran Reformation in 1536.[45] As underlined in Chapter 2, most of the medieval sources in Northern Europe relating to health care and poor relief detail positive events, such as the disposition of 1175 of abbot William of Æbelholt monastery, referred to by Thomas Riis, which instituted an annual mass for the abbot on his death-day and ordained a special meal or feast for the friars of Æbelholt commemorating him, while twelve poor – note the symbolic and apostolic number – were to receive a free meal on that day. In this connection it is noteworthy that in the 700 or so foundation-letters of masses for the dead issued between 1460 and 1540, only between a third and a ninth of their total donations went towards the assistance of the lay poor while the rest was allocated for the church and religious purposes.[46] By their nature such medieval documents distinguish themselves from most of the post-Reformation sources, which are administrative in origin and accordingly tend to focus on shortcomings and plans for improvement.

The Reformation of Denmark and Norway followed a four-year-long civil war, which proved disruptive and costly. This obviously made it extremely difficult to fulfill the intentions laid down in the new Protestant Church Order of 1537, which had been formulated under the supervision of Johannes Bugenhagen. It may well have been the social and economic effects of this internal strife which was the cause of the increased incidence of begging in the country, rather than the disruptions caused by the demolition of the Catholic Church and its system of alms collection and distribution. Undoubtedly the new Lutheran welfare system needed time before it could work properly. Inexperience and confusion would to some extent have contributed to these difficulties, but most important of all would have been the economic constraints the new system had to be introduced under. The economic resources, which the new overseers of the poor took over from their clerical, Catholic predecessors, often proved inadequate and for years remained under constant legal threat from donors' families who sought to repossess land which had been donated for the benefit of both the involuntary poor and the Catholic Church. With the abolition of masses for the dead and vigils, at least part of the original contract could be claimed to have been broken. In this situation only the unflinching support of the Lutheran king Christian III guaranteed that most of the original resources were retained for the lay poor.[47]

Initially the Reformation only resulted in the magistracies in the major towns and cities taking over the larger urban monasteries and turning them into hospitals for the local poor and sick, while the larger rural monasteries were allowed gradually to be run down over a generation or more while continuing to offer hostelry to poor travellers, until their final desolution in the 1580s and 90s. The Reformation in Denmark, like the reforms in health care and poor relief, was in other words a gradual affair which was only entering its finishing stages at the beginning of the seventeenth century. Acordingly most of the medieval hospitals or houses of the Holy

Spirit were allowed to continue after the Reformation, as pointed out by Riis. But they continued with a significant difference – namely as purely lay institutions geared to the needs of the involuntary, lay poor.

That both indoor relief in hospitals and outdoor relief in a large measure continued to depend on alms collecting throughout the sixteenth century, despite the Reformation, can hardly surprise. Evidently the pressure from a growing and impoverished population put the available resources under strain. The newly instituted collections after church services were obviously unable to cover the shortfall, and organised collections by licensed collectors proved necessary. But as opposed to alms gathering by the mendicant orders before the Reformation, these organised collections were for purely lay purposes and intended exclusively for the lay involuntary poor and sick.

The ambition to create new and larger district hospitals in the 1540s, catering for the poor and elderly as well as the sick, was a more or less direct consequence of the Reformation. For a number of reasons it never proved an unmitigated success. The financial resources available often proved inadequate, while many local communities were unwilling to contribute economically to hospitals over which they had little or no influence. Consequently in 1558 the government changed its hospital policy and returned to a structure where most market towns were allowed their own hospital.

For the Reformation king, Christian III, it was a natural obligation of a good and godly government to provide its subjects with medical care, especially outside the capital Copenhagen where trained medical men were hard to find. Thus the king authorised his royal physician Cornelius Hamsfort to open a pharmacy in Odense in 1549, granting him a house in the city, free of tax and with a monopoly on the production of drugs. Christian III had taken this initiative because he had realised that 'there was a severe shortage of physicians and good apothecaries in his kingdom which caused many of the king's subjects and visitors to these parts to die of neglect when they fell ill'.[48]

The religious confrontation between Catholics and Protestants which surrounded the outbreak of the Thirty Years' War and characterised this war until the early 1630s, created an apocalyptic and millenarian mood within European Protestantism.[49] In Denmark these apocalyptic sentiments became closely linked to the disastrous intervention in the Thirty Years' War by the Danish king Christian IV. It resulted in a religiously based programme of welfare reform, initiated primarily from the centre, but fully supported by many localities, as pointed out by Ladewig Petersen.[50]

However, even before his failed attempt to lead the Protestant camp to victory in the Thirty Years' War, Christian IV had taken the opportunity to provide his capital with a number of social institutions, which like so much of the king's programme for urban renewal was inspired by similar institutions in the United Provinces.[51] Thus in 1605 the king had established a house of correction in Copenhagen, followed in 1619 by an orphanage. Considering the cost to the government of these two institutions – at least 8,000 thalers annually in the 1640s – which housed between 300 to 500 inmates, the mercantilist rationale behind these institutions may not have been so clear cut. That the orphans and criminals should be employed 'for His Royal Majesty's profit' may well refer to a much broader Protestant and utilitarian motive: namely to train and employ such people so that they might become useful and contributing individuals to the Christian commonwealth.

The re-organisation and reform of poor relief in Copenhagen in 1630, following the defeat in the Thirty Years' War, was introduced in honour of God and for the solace of the poor. Begging was forbidden. Instead the deserving poor were to receive quarterly alms from the overseers, whose funds depended partly on the interest of 60,000 thalers, voluntary gifts and church collections. That Christian IV should have initially limited his reforms to Copenhagen is hardly surprising. Poverty was undoubtedly most prominent in the by then fast growing capital, where the king resided and which remained the focus for so many of his initiatives. However, the scheme was copied by some of the larger provincial towns such as Ribe and Odense and possibly by Viborg where a centralisation of the diverse resources took place. Where the Copenhagen reforms depended wholly on voluntary contributions, the system adopted in Ribe of annual contributions from the town's merchants appears to have been something of a halfway house between a tax and a system of voluntary donations. In Odense, however, Christian IV took the opportunity to introduce an annual poor rate. The reforms made sums available for these three towns which would have made it possible for the authorities to maintain around 2–4 per cent of the population.[52] These figures appear to be at the lower end compared with the number of dependant poor in

the urban centres of Europe where the authorities generally seem to
have been able to make alms available for at least 5 per cent of the
population.[53]

As Ladewig Petersen points out, it is remarkable that the crown's
contributions towards charity and education peaked in the late
1580s at a time when private charity began to grow dramatically.
First of all it demonstrates that the post-Reformation governments
considered a welfare policy an essential part of its religious and
political programme for which it was willing to provide substantial
funds. That private charity proved slow in expanding may well have
depended on two factors. First, it took time for the country and its
citizens to recuperate from the economic and social disruption of the
civil war of the 1530s, while the benefits of the general European
economic boom of the second half of the sixteenth century, which
had witnessed a growing demand for Danish agricultural products,
did not filter through to the nobility, clergy and leading burghers
until the 1580s. Second, the changes generated by the Reformation
took time to become an organic and accepted feature in the many
localities where this private charity blossomed from the 1580s until
the end of the Thirty Years' War.[54]

SWEDEN

As in Denmark, the impact of the Reformation proved significant
for the transformation of health care and poor relief which took
place in Sweden and Finland during the sixteenth- and seventeenth
centuries, as E. I. Kouri emphasises.[55] In the crown's general
takeover of the patrimony of the Catholic Church, which began in
1527, Gustav Vasa took special measures to safeguard those
institutions which had been predominantly geared toward charity,
such as the houses and hospitals of the Holy Spirit. The king
repeatedly intervened to protect these institutions from the
encroachment of private individuals, who sought to regain land
and donations given by their ancestors now that these institutions
no longer fulfilled the spiritual service, such as masses for the dead,
as originally specified in the letters of foundation.

Thus it was the Swedish reformer Olaus Petri who formulated the
Stockholm Statute of 1533 which the magistracy introduced and the
king approved. This statute created the basis for a reform of
hospitals not only in the capital, but eventually in most of the major
towns in Sweden and Finland. Apart from the traditional detailed

Protestant provisions for the administration of the hospitals, and rules of admission which specified that only the seriously ill or elderly incapable of looking after themselves were to be admitted into the hospitals, the Stockholm Statute encouraged cleanliness, emphasising that the inmates were to bathe regularly, and underlined the need for a physician to be appointed to attend residents.

The Stockholm Hospital of the Holy Spirit continued to cater for a number of paying pensioners, the so-called 'free brethren', after the Reformation, but their number may well have fallen substantially *vis-à-vis* the sick and poor. Thus in 1557 only a quarter of the inmates were pensioners. Four years later when the hospital had moved to more hygienic and presumably larger premises in Danviken, since the number of inmates grew from 98 to 160, the proportion of pensioners had fallen to 7 per cent.

Poor relief in Sweden and Finland, however, continued to be parish-based after the Reformation and the church continued to be responsible for its collection and administration through the newly created poor boxes or common chests. Charity in the first generation after the Reformation, indoor as well as outdoor, depended to a large extent on royal donations. Only slowly did the effects of prolonged warfare and repeated rebellions fade away and make more resources available locally. By then, however, the welfare system had come under pressure from a growing population which saw the number of destitute increase dramatically.

Throughout the late sixteenth- and seventeenth century central government tried to deal with these problems by ordering local communities to look after their own resident poor; rural parishes were admonished not to encourage their poor to seek support in the nearest urban centres where resources were already over-extended. Instead they were repeatedly instructed to establish their own small almshouses or infirmaries as a supplement to the larger diocesan hospitals. In spite of repeated attempts from the centre to establish a network of small local infirmaries on the periphery, these government initiatives had only produced patchy results by the end of the seventeenth century.

Gutavus Adolphus attempted a further re-organisation of health care and poor relief in 1619 when he proposed a scheme for improving the financial basis for indoor relief by enlarging and centralising the diocesan hospitals in Sweden and Finland. The clergy in particular, however, proved unreceptive to the king's idea

that the local parishes should contribute to these larger institutions
in accordance with the number of inmates or patients originating
from their communities. Increased poverty and begging made the
king realise that something had to be done urgently, and in 1624
legislation was passed which outlawed begging and created the legal
framework for an amalgamation of existing hospitals, reducing
them from twenty-one to eleven, thereby increasing the number of
inmates they could cater for while simultaneously ridding them of
those who were perceived to be idlers and work-shy. Workhouses
were to be established for such undeserving poor in all the
provinces, while inmates or patients in the centralised hospitals had
to pay an admission fee. It was envisaged that these reforms were to
be financed by an annual tax or poor rate. These ambitious plans,
however, proved impossible to implement. Only some moderate
reforms took place in urban centres such as Stockholm, while a
military hospital was established in the former monastery of
Vadstena in 1638. Considering Sweden's leading military role in the
Thirty Years' War, the creation of such an institution was hardly
surprising. But the grand design for a network of workhouses and
orphanages across the country financed by a poor rate was never
implemented.

Later, in 1642, the government indirectly acknowledged that its
1624 programme had been over-ambitious. The poor relief order of
1642 allowed regulated and licensed begging. Gone were the grand
plans for large-scale institutions which would deal with indoor
relief, instead the government once more returned to the well tested
system of parish relief, encouraging these communities to construct
poorhouses linked to the local churches. It was only four years earlier
that Stockholm had finally acquired a combined workhouse and
orphanage, and the city remained unique in Sweden throughout the
seventeenth century in having such an institution.

Once more, however, it proved difficult to implement even these
limited reforms, especially in Stockholm where poverty and begging
was endemic. In 1663 the magistracy re-issued an extended version
of the poor order of 1642. A poor rate was introduced in the city and
collected by a group of officially appointed collectors. Outside of
Stockholm, major reforms of the welfare system introduced in the
decades after the Reformation proved impossible to implement in
the provinces. A few local reforms, however, met with some success,
such as those introduced by the Bishop of Åbo, Johannes Gezelius
the younger, who in 1699 had the parishioners in his diocese draw

up a list of the resident deserving poor whom local residents were obliged to support according to their financial ability. This system became a forerunner for the rote system of relief which allocated individual poor to be maintained by one or more local farms. Eventually this approach became the cornerstone of poor relief in eighteenth-century Sweden and Finland.[56]

DANZIG

The Reformation proved important for the welfare reforms which were likewise introduced in Danzig during the second half of the sixteenth century, as emphasised by Maria Bogucka. The two poor laws of 1525 and 1551 in the main sought to regulate and control begging, which as in most other European cities of this period had increasingly become a nuisance. Furthermore, in the 1550s, the magistracy created a centralised charity board, the *Spendeamt*, to administer all of Danzig's welfare schemes, outdoor as well as indoor relief, in the city's nine hospitals. Undoubtedly the welfare reforms of the 1550s are closely linked to the fact that this was exactly the period when the Reformation was officially established and the *Confessio Augustana* formally recognised in Royal Prussia. That further reforms in the welfare domain were taken by the city authorities in 1606 and 1610 should be seen in the context of the victory of Lutheran orthodoxy in Danzig during these years which brought to an end a period of tolerant Protestant co-existence and resulted in the expulsion of non-Lutheran Protestants.[57]

Indoor relief in Danzig was, as in most other cities in Northern Europe, offered through the city's hospitals, which catered for the traditional mixture of elderly pensioners, the poor, invalid and sick. Only the smallpox hospital and the plague hospital appear to have been exclusively geared to treating and nursing the sick. Danzig appears to have been unusually early in establishing an orphanage in 1542 – a decade before Antwerp, and a couple of generations before most of the other cities discussed in this volume. How and why this came about is difficult to explain. While the orphanages in Antwerp may well have been encouraged by the considerable Italian immigrant population in the city who were well acquainted with institutions such as the *Ospedale degli Innocenti* in leading Italian cities such as Florence and Venice, the source of inspiration in Danzig is less obvious.[58]

The workhouse established in Danzig in 1629 was clearly

inspired by earlier developments in the Dutch Republic. Similar lines of influence are, however, less obvious when it comes to the medical regulatory body, the *Collegium Medicum*, which Danzig acquired in 1636, coinciding with the creation of a similar body in Amsterdam, but which Antwerp, by then a Catholic city, had acquired sixteen years earlier.[59] Most central governments as well as the magistracies in the majority of major Northern European cities appear to have been preoccupied with the need for regulation and control of the growing number of medical services which were becoming available to the population during the early seventeenth century. If the city in question possessed a university the control and regulation tended to fall to the professors of the medical faculty, as can seen from the medical regulation for Copenhagen issued in 1619, rather than a *Collegium Medicum*, which initially appears only to have been created in cities which possessed no university.[60]

ENGLAND

In his chapter dealing with London, apart from Paris the fastest growing and by far the largest city in Northern Europe by the beginning of the seventeenth century, Paul Slack charts five chronological phases in the development of the capital's hospitals and workhouses, which he labels the royal, the civic, the metropolitan, the baroque and the voluntary period.[61] The restoration and foundation of five London hospitals in the reign of Edward VI for the sick, the old, the upbringing and education of orphans, the lunatics, and the old royal palace at Bridewell as a workhouse, was closely linked to the young monarch's Protestant faith and desire for reform. Simultaneously a centralisation of all health care and poor relief in London was undertaken on a par with most continental cities where the Reformation had been victorious. All indoor and outdoor relief was to be centrally administered for the whole city, even if collections were still to be conducted within the framework of the parish. As Slack points out, some of the inspiration for this reform may well have come from the foreign communities in London who had just been granted a royal charter allowing them to establish their own Dutch and Walloon-French Reformed churches in the city, and whose deep commitment to Christian charity later generated widespread admiration within the host community. Considering how close the leader of the foreign churches, Johannes à Lasco, was to Archbishop Thomas Cranmer, staying with him at Lambeth Palace for most of 1550, this seems a reasonable assumption.[62] The strangers, whose ecclesiastical ideal was the Reformed Church of Zurich, would at least have caused their hosts to look in that direction. The Bishop of London, Nicholas Ridley, who strongly supported the hospital reforms, brings to mind Zwingli's repeated reference to the involuntary poor as 'living images of God' when, commenting on the reforms he stated that 'Christ should lie no more abroad in the streets'.[63] A further source of inspiration, equally close to home and to the foreign Reformed churches in London, may have been the reformer Martin Bucer who had arrived in England from Strasburg in 1549 and been given the Regius Chair in Divinity at Cambridge.[64]

Furthermore, many of the English merchants who had resided in Antwerp where the Merchant Adventurers had their staple until 1564, may well have been impressed by the reforms of poor relief which had taken place in neighbouring Ypres and Bruges a couple of decades earlier, and may have wanted to see similar reforms realised at home.[65] Such aspirations may well have been furthered by visitors such as Andreas Hyperius, who, as already mentioned, had stayed in England between 1537 and 1541 and whose tract on the reform of poor relief was later to be translated into English.

Undoubtedly the high-profile Dutch welfare institutions of the late sixteenth- and seventeenth century proved highly influential in most of Western Europe, but not all of them were specifically Dutch inventions. The famous Amsterdam workhouse – the *rasphuis* – which opened up in 1596 was actually an English innovation and was inspired by the workhouses created first at Bridewell in London in 1552 and later in Norwich. Once more the presence of the Dutch and Walloon foreign communities in London and in Norwich, where the refugees constituted around a third of the population towards the end of the sixteenth century, appears to have been of considerable significance. Many of these refugees retained close contacts with their home country and later returned to Holland and Zeeland in the 1590s when the Dutch revolt was on a secure footing and a strong economic upturn had become clearly identifiable, and they are most likely to have served as intermediaries, bringing the concept of the workhouse back with them to the United Provinces.[66]

The need for a workhouse – *tuichthuis* – in the rapidly expanding city of Amsterdam appears to have been realised within the Amsterdam magistracy by 1589, and they may well have commissioned one of their fellow councillors Jan Laurensz Spiegel to write a memorandum on the foundation of a *tuichthuis*. Spiegel proposed that a workhouse should be established in the former Clarissa convent which had been confiscated by the city council. It should be converted in order to prevent inmates from escaping and made suitable for the installation of workshops. The aim of this house of correction was not simply to punish criminals and disorderlies, but to improve and reform the way of life of those who did not realise the value to them of such an institution.

The incarceration of such people should not be undertaken in order to brand them publicly, but should serve to turn them into valuable citizens. The inmates should be transformed into healthy and industrious individuals who wanted to work and to contribute to the commonwealth and, last but not least, to become God-fearing. To avoid stigmatisation of the inmates, their sentences were to be handed out *in camera* while their commitment should happen under the cover of darkness. No visitors were to be allowed and the officials involved in their imprisonment had to take an oath promising not to reveal their identities.[67] Seven years later the Amsterdam *rasphuis* situated in the converted Clarissa convent was ready to receive its first prisoners, and an institution which was to be much admired by visitors to the city over the next century had come into existence. The example of Amsterdam inspired other cities and Haarlem, Gouda, Enkhuizen, Alkmaar and Dordrecht quickly followed suit.

The founders' ambition to re-educate destitute beggars and criminals and turn them into pious and hard-working citizens proved futile, and undoubtedly explains why these institutions did not proliferate further. Instead, the penal element gradually took over and most of the inmates appear to have become long-term residents.[68] This was certainly the case at Bridewell in London, and in 1582 the Privy Council found it necessary to stipulate that this institution had been established for the 'reformation' of the poor. Accordingly, they were expected to stay for a short term only and not, as the Privy Council put it, perpetually.[69]

It is not only the hospital reforms in the reign of Edward VI which prove the Protestant antecedents of the welfare reforms introduced in England in the sixteenth- and seventeenth centuries. In the 1530s two projects for the relief and employment of the poor were put forward by the Protestant printer and translator William Marshall, who was responsible for translating the order for the reform of poor relief in Ypres into English, and the anticlerical common lawyer Christopher St German, who later became a major source of inspiration for the Leveller leader John Lilburne.[70] St German may not have been a Protestant by strict theological criteria, but he was considered a major enemy of the Catholic Church by Thomas More. Possessing one of the best legal minds of the age, St German forced More to concede that the councils of the church could err, and he argued that the church was bound by the canonical Scriptures accepted by the early church.[71]

Later in Elizabeth's reign major Protestant figures within the government took the lead in the practical and legislative reforms of poor relief which took place, in particular Sir Francis Walsingham and William Cecil, Lord Burghley, while Walsingham together with another two Reformed peers, Robert Dudley, Earl of Leicester, and Henry Hastings, Earl of Huntingdon, were directly involved in local schemes for welfare reform in Oxford, Warwick and Winchester.[72]

Kett's rebellion in 1549 appears to have encouraged the first local steps towards the English Poor Law of 1598. Voluntary parochial collections were replaced in Norwich in 1549 and in York in 1550 with compulsory levies for the poor. These examples from the periphery encouraged Parliament to move in the same direction a couple of years later when a statute was issued which still retained the voluntary principle but ordered weekly church collections to be held while condemning begging.

The next social and political rebellion – the Rising in the North of 1569 – caused central government as well as local authorities to take further action. In 1570 in Norwich it may have led to a census of the poor, schemes for their employment and the education of poor children to be introduced, and a workhouse on a par with Bridewell to be created at Acle. Under its Puritan mayor John Aldrich and with its large immigrant population of Dutch and Walloon Calvinists, this Reformed stronghold not only took the lead locally, but also played a significant part in inspiring the parliamentary legislation which followed in 1572 – Aldrich had become an MP in this year, while the Norwich initiatives had attracted the attention of Archbishop Matthew Parker.[73] The Act of 1572 introduced for the first time a compulsory poor rate. The Justices of the Peace should take regular surveys of the poor and assess and tax the inhabitants of their county in order to provide for the needy. They were also instructed to appoint overseers of the poor in each parish who should inspect the local poor on a monthly basis, in order to make sure that vagrants and undeserving poor were excluded from the dole. Houses of correction were to be established in every county and stocks of raw materials should be made available in order to put the unemployed to work.

In practice, however, the 1572 act fell well short of what was intended. The workhouses which were established proved far from adequate to deal with the growing number of vagrants, the Justices of the Peace were unable to cope with the considerable new administrative obligations placed on their shoulders, while overseers refused to accept their appointments and many parishioners refused to pay the rates.

It took another crisis to generate further action. The harvest failures of the 1590s and the threatening grain riots once more brought welfare reforms back on top of the parliamentary agenda in the winter of 1597–8. Many of the leading figures on the parliamentary committees considering new social reforms and regulations were prominent Puritans, such as the Essex gentleman Sir Robert Wroth.[74] In other words, the driving forces behind the legislation of 1598 were, as had been the case with the earlier initiatives, committed Protestants.

The Vagrancy and Poor Relief statutes of 1598 established the three fundamentals of the English Poor Law to which further legislation of the early seventeenth century only added details. First, vagrants were to be punished and workhouses were to be created in all major towns and in all counties. Second, outdoor relief was to be financed by poor rates. This system became commonplace in the generation after 1598, and by 1624 poor rates were universal in the larger towns and gradually becoming common in the more populous rural parishes. The responsibility for the collection of the rates fell to the churchwardens and overseers of the poor in each parish, who were also responsible for the distribution of alms to the deserving poor. Third, work was to be provided for the able-bodied poor. This last element proved the most difficult to implement and most churchwardens appear to have preferred payments in cash to such poor rather than having to arrange and supervise the work of the unemployed.[75]

The Poor Law undoubtedly provided England with an impressive public welfare system which was unique in early modern Northern Europe, even if its dependence on the parish and the annual assessments made it somewhat inflexible and slow in responding to major crises such as serious outbreaks of plague. Two questions, however, spring to mind in this context. First, how different were the English poor rates, built on local assessment, from subscriptions or door-to-door collections and weekly collections at the church door in the period we are concerned with? Perhaps the English poor rates have tended to be seen as too similar to twentieth-century taxes by historians conditioned by Western European societies obsessed with taxation. Second, why did England manage successfully to introduce a poor rate, while as we shall see, it was only contemplated in Germany, Sweden and the Spanish Netherlands, and introduced in one or two towns in Denmark, while in Scotland where it was introduced in the 1570s, it only seems to have been implemented in a couple of the more important burghs, as pointed out by Rosalind Mitchison?[76]

With regard to the first question it may well be the case that the actual difference between rates and door-to-door collections were minimal in the early modern period. The assessment of rates by your local equals or peers would in practice have come close to the subscription system used in collections among the membership by many Reformed communities in the early seventeenth century and later in the century in England by the Society for the Promoting of Christian Knowledge, decribed by Paul Slack in what he terms the voluntary episode. The example of the practice of the Dutch Reformed community in London may serve to illustrate this point. Whenever the regular weekly collections by the deacons at the church door of Austin Friars proved inadequate, door-to-door collections were initiated. A look at the collection lists preserved from these collections, some incomplete and therefore most revealing in this context, show that the amounts expected to be collected were determined by the wealthier and in most cases leading members of the church, signing first for the sums they were to donate, thereby setting a certain standard for each collection and for what lesser members were expected to give. This appears to have been a semi-public system, thus serving to put moral and social pressure on the general membership to follow suit and donate the sums expected of them.[77] This was in other words a flexible system which came close to a poor rate.

But that still leaves us with the question of why England managed successfully to introduce a poor rate in the late sixteenth- and early seventeenth centuries at a time when other countries failed. An explanation may well be found in the protracted character of the

English Reformation, starting with what might well be termed the royal phase which in the social sphere included the hospital reforms and central administration of welfare provisions introduced in the reign of Edward VI, followed by the interplay between centre and periphery which characterised the Elizabethan period, not only in terms of social policy which led to the Poor Relief Statutes of 1598, but also in religion, with constant attempts from Calvinists or Puritans to force the Anglican Church and the Elizabethan government further down the road of reform.[78] This process continued well into the 1650s when it finally ran out of steam. This long Reformation carried within it a special dynamic which repeatedly served to inspire new generations of Protestants and which, together with the dramatic growth of London during this period, may well have encouraged government and Parliament to press with far greater determination for the creation of a poor rate than was the case in the rest of Northern Europe in the early modern period.

In the reigns of James I and Charles I a considerable and growing number of Reformed Protestants found themselves at odds with the government and the Church of England. Proposals for welfare reforms, however, continued to be forthcoming from godly Protestants, such as Sir Thomas Middleton, President of Bridewell, who in 1623 proposed a parish-based scheme for smaller workhouses in London, where the poor should be involved in manufacture using hemp and flax. Middleton was a leading London merchant who had resided in Antwerp before returning to London in 1582. Upon his return he became a member of the Dutch Reformed Church in the city, and when becoming Lord Mayor of London in 1613 he requested the Dutch community to include him in their regular Sunday prayer where reference should be made only to a 'brother' who was about to take on a burdensome public office.[79]

Sir Thomas Middleton's scheme was later incorporated into the great Puritan welfare scheme, the Corporation of the Poor, which was established in London between 1647 and 1649. This was a scheme which sought to re-introduce some of the elements of centralisation of poor relief originally included in the Edwardian reforms of the previous century. This project was vigorously supported by Samuel Hartlib and his friends, among them a prominent merchant and member of the Dutch Reformed community in the city, Nicolas Corselis, who also served among the governing assistants of the London Corporation after 1649.[80]

The urgent need for new social relief agencies in London during the Civil War, where traditional avenues of relief were breaking down due to the pressures of an ill-fed population which had been swelled by a considerable influx of destitute migrants and wounded soldiers, helped bring about the creation of the Corporation of the Poor while inspiring a number of tracts on welfare reforms from staunch Calvinist and Puritan controversalists.[81] Among them was the physician Peter Chamberlen who, like his Huguenot father and uncle, was a committed Protestant who specialised in midwifery. In the late 1640s, having recently returned from a brief exile in the Netherlands, Chamberlen appears to have personally employed an apothecary at his house and offered free medical and midwifery assistance to the poor. He considered medicine and health measures an essential part of public poor relief, as can be seen from his tract on social welfare published in 1649, *The Poore Mans Advocate*.[82] Here he argued that church lands should be confiscated to finance the settlement of poor families, who in return for their labour would be provided with free medical services including hospitals.

Chamberlen's writings expressed views similar to those already promoted by the attorney John Cook, who defended John Lilburne before the House of Lords and became Solicitor-General in 1649, acting as public prosecutor at the trial of Charles I. Cook had published his arguments for welfare reforms in 1648 under the title *Unum Necessarium; or, The Poore Mans Case: Being an Expedient to make Provision for All Poor People in the Kingdome*. His tract was unusual in more than one respect. He argued that physicians and attorneys should do a tenth of their work for the poor without receiving any fees, and he was probably the first writer to make a direct association between poverty and criminality, suggesting that convicted criminals should be given a second chance.[83]

It is, however, his concern for health care and medical provision for the poor which is the most prominent feature of *The Poore Mans Case*. Local government was expected to alleviate the dangers of malnutrition and hunger among the poor by introducing price controls on grain, but Cook realised that preventative measures would not provide full protection against disease. The cost of consulting physicians and paying apothecaries' bills were, according to Cook, beyond the means of the poor. Furthermore, many market towns did not possess a resident physician. Consequently, Cook advocated total deregulation of the medical market, allowing all able practitioners to offer their services, and he encouraged the local clergy to aquire some medical knowledge and take on medical responsibilities so that they could assist the sick poor. Furthermore, Cook wanted some form of basic medical training to be given to the poor themselves in areas where no medical assistance was available, in order to make it possible for them to produce some simple drugs for their own use.

By far the most detailed and wide-ranging proposal for reform of contemporary health care provision was put forward by William Petty, a Samuel Hartlib associate, in his *The Advice of W. P. to Mr. Samuel Hartlib*, which was also published in 1648. Petty had received his medical education in the Dutch Republic, where he had matriculated at the University of Leiden in May 1644. Here he would have benefited from the clinical or bedside teaching recently introduced by Otto Heurnius and developed by the Huguenot immigrant Franciscus de la Boë Sylvius, who also gave lessons in anatomy in Leiden.[84] It was undoubtedly his experience of clinical medicine in Leiden and Utrecht which inspired Petty's elaborate plan for a teaching hospital which he advocated in his *Advice*. Petty saw such an institution as developing out of one of the 'old Hospitals'. He thought this could be achieved without much extra cost, since the staff would be no larger than normal and their salaries should not be excessive. He envisaged the hospital to have a staff of unmarried men who would be dedicated to public service.

The teaching hospital was to be administered by a board of four. The day-to-day running of this institution should fall to a 'Steward', preferably a mathematician with knowledge of accounting and architecture who could also assist the medical personnel by investigating astrology and medical statistics. The medical staff should be led by a 'Physician', a leading figure within his 'profession' who was skilled in classical as well as modern medicine, and who would conduct dissections and prepare alchemical remedies. This senior physician would supervise his colleagues and educate junior personnel while visiting all patients in the hospital twice a day. He was to be helped by a 'Vice-physician' who would be responsible for the clinical study and the compilation of case histories. A number of medical students would work within the hospital and each receive a salary of twenty-five pounds. They would help not only the physicians, but also the surgeons, apothecaries and even the nurses. Having worked and studied within the hospital for five years the medical students – only four years were needed for surgeons' and apothecaries' apprentices – would be issued with certificates permitting them to practise wherever they wanted.[85] Petty's plans appear, in part at least, to have been realised in the two nationalised London hospitals, Ely House and the Savoy, which were initially established in the 1640s solely for military purposes. But their existence proved fairly shortlived. They were abolished at the Restoration and the clinical teaching which had begun there did not become commonplace in London until the end of the seventeenth century.[86]

SCOTLAND

In contrast with the rest of Northern Europe, where the Reformation and Protestantism proved of such paramount importance for the range and speed of the welfare reforms in this period, Scotland presents a totally different picture. As Rosalind Mitchison points out, little if anything was achieved in Scotland in the sixteenth- and seventeenth centuries despite the fact that a poor law modelled on the English Act of 1572 was introduced in the late 1570s. Even though social reforms were part of the Reformation which the Scottish reformer John Knox had envisaged, and the Book of Discipline of 1560 had proposed that part of the patrimony of the Catholic Church be used to support the poor, hardly anything was achieved.[87]

This was largely due to two factors. First, there was very little pre-Reformation Catholic welfare structure to build on in Scotland. Second, and more importantly, the Scottish Reformation was not linked to the emergence of strong territorial or urban government as in the rest of Northern Europe. Instead, it was closely linked to the political struggle for power within the Scottish feudal elite. As opposed to other countries where the Reformation was victorious, Scotland possessed not only a weak central government, but also a local government which remained feeble until 1660.[88] Consequently it took considerable time for the Reformed Church to establish itself in the country and only slowly did a proper church structure with ministers and elders come into existence; thus by 1600 many northern parishes in the Lowlands had still to receive a minister.

Furthermore, Scotland was a large and in many parts impassable country with only a small and generally poor population, which in itself made it difficult to govern. Not surprisingly the Scottish Poor Law of the 1570s only had some impact in a few of the more important towns or burghs and, as Mitchison emphasises, the government never made any serious attempt to try to introduce it in the countryside where 90 per cent of the population lived.

Despite the new Poor Law Act of 1592 which stipulated that parish officials responsible for poor relief should be appointed, nothing happened in Scotland. By then a poor rate had become a permanent feature only in Edinburgh, not least as a consequence of the serious outbreak of plague in 1584, and gradually it was introduced in some of the major urban areas such as St Andrews in 1597, Perth in 1599, Aberdeen in 1619, and in Glasgow and Dundee in 1636. But not even the serious harvest failures of 1622–3 which caused many peasants to leave their land in search of food could convince local authorities to introduce some form of rate. When the Privy Council ordered a temporary poor rate to be raised to avoid a national famine many parishes angrily refused to cooperate.

It is noteworthy that in 1649, when the poor law had finally become effective in most Lowland parishes, a revitalised Reformed movement represented by the Covenanting Party had already been in power for more than a decade and probably played a considerable part in its introduction.[89] Thus Protestantism in an unusually delayed form may well have helped along the welfare reforms in Scotland towards the middle of the seventeenth century even if real improvement in poor relief had to wait until the eighteenth century.

Some medical care for the sick poor, however, seems to have been available in the major towns by the early seventeenth century, when Edinburgh appointed a surgeon to attend the poor on a regular basis and Glasgow introduced a system of care which became permanent in the 1650s.

Rosalind Mitchison's concluding statement, telling us not to ask why societies generally ignored the needs of the poor and failed to provide them with relief, but rather why in some periods they did manage to take some action, may serve as a fitting epilogue for this volume. Something, even if it may be considered limited and inadequate from a modern perspective, was done to improve health care provision and poor relief in early modern Northern Europe, and the range and speed of these welfare reforms would not have been imaginable without the Reformation.

NOTES

1   See P. Slack, *Poverty and Policy in Tudor and Stuart England*, London 1988; P. Slack, *The Impact of Plague in Tudor and Stuart England*, London 1985; R. M. Smith (ed.) *Land, Kinship and Life-Cycle*, Cambridge 1984; M. Pelling and R. M. Smith (eds) *Life, Death and the Elderly: historical perspectives*, London 1991; M. Pelling, 'Healing the Sick Poor: social policy and disability in Norwich 1550–1640', *Medical History*, 29, 1985; C. Webster, *The Great Instauration: science, medicine and reform 1626–60*, London 1975; C. Webster (ed.) *Health, Medicine and Mortality in the Sixteenth Century*, Cambridge 1979.

2   See also J. Barry and C. Jones (eds) *Medicine and Charity Before the Welfare State*, London 1991, especially the introduction, 1–13 and S. Cavallo, 'The Motivations of Benefactors: an overview of approaches to the study of charity', 46–62.

3   See Chapter 5 of this volume.

4   A. Wear, 'Caring for the Sick Poor in St Bartholomew's Exchange: 1580–1676', in R. Porter and W. Bynum (eds) 'Living and Dying in London', *Medical History*, Supplement 11, 1991, 41–60. See also Chapter 5 of this volume.

5   See O. P. Grell, 'The Religious Duty of Care and the Social Need for Control in Early Modern Europe', *Historical Journal*, 39, 1996, 257–63; and Chapter 2 of this volume.

6   See Chapter 2 of this volume.

7   See L. Palmer Wandel, 'Social Welfare', in H. J. Hillerbrand (ed.) *The Oxford Encyclopedia of the Reformation*, New York 1996, 4, 77–83; and Chapter 2 of this volume.

8   See A. T. van Deursen, *Bavianen en Slijkgeusen. Kerk en Kerkvolk ten tijde van Maurits en Oldenbarnevelt*, Franeker 1991, 115.

9   A. J. Jelsma and O. Boersma (eds) *Acta van het Consistorie van de Nederlandse Gemeente te Londen 1569–1585*, Rijks Geschiedkundige Publicatiën uitgegeven door het Instituut voor Nederlandse Geschiedenis, Kleine Serie 76, The Hague 1993, 526–7.

10   *ibid.*, 387–8.

11   See Deursen, *Bavianen en Slijkgeusen*, 115, 123; for London, see *Acta . . . van de Nederlandse Gemeente te Londen*, 279.

12   See Guildhall Library, London, MS 7397/8, fol. 20v.

13   Deusen, *Bavianen en Slijkgeusen*, 104–6; for the Dutch Revolt, see J. I. Israel, *The Dutch Republic: its rise, greatness, and fall, 1477–806*, Oxford 1995.

14   R. B. Evenhuis, *Ook dat was Amsterdam. De kerk der hervorming in de gouden eeuw*, Amsterdam 1967, vol. 2, 76.

15   Deursen, *Bavianen en Slijkgeusen*, 117–23.

16   Guildhall Library, London, MS 7424, f.9; for Archbishop Laud and the foreign churches in England, see O. P. Grell, *Dutch Calvinists in Early Stuart London*, Leiden 1989, 224–48.

17   See Chapter 3 of this volume.

18   See Chapter 11 of this volume.

19 See A. Pettegree, *Foreign Protestant Communities in Sixteenth-Century London*, Oxford 1986, 203.
20 Grell, *Dutch Calvinists*, 99–100; for Lancelot Andrewes's observation, see C. Hill, 'Puritans and the Poor', *Past and Present*, 2, 1952, 44.
21 See A. A. Van Schelven (ed.) *Kerkeraads-Protocollen der Nederduitsche Vluchtelingen-Kerk te Londen*, Amsterdam 1921, 428–35; see also O. P. Grell, 'Plague in Elizabethan and Stuart London: the Dutch response', *Medical History*, 34, 1990, 424–39, especially 426–7. As in the case of the Dutch Church in London, the position of visitor of the sick in the United Provinces appears to have been created as a result of outbreaks of plague: in Amsterdam in 1589, in Leiden in 1595, and in Rotterdam in 1596; see Deursen, *Bavianen en Slijkgeusen*, 99.
22 See Grell, 'Plague in London', 427; and M. J. van Lieburg, 'Geneeskundige Zorg als Kerkelijke Taak. De situatie in de gereformeerde kerk van Rotterdam in de zeventiende eeuw', in *De Zeventiende Eeuw*, 1989, 5,1, 162–71.
23 *Acta... van de Nederlandse Gemeente te Londen*, 71 and 73–4; see also O. Boersma, *Vluchtig Voorbeeld. De Nederlandse, Franse en Italiaanse vluchtelingenkerken in Londen, 1568–85*, Kampen 1994, 122–3.
24 Grell, 'Plague in London', 431–5; see also O. P. Grell, 'Conflicting Duties: plague and the obligations of early modern physicians towards patients and commonwealth in England and the Netherlands', in A. Wear *et al.*, *Doctors and Ethics: the earlier historical setting of professional ethics*, Amsterdam 1993, 131–52, especially 139; and Deursen, *Bavianen en Slijkgeusen*, 98–101.
25 For this, see A. Pettegree, *Emden and the Dutch Revolt: exile and the development of Reformed Protestantism*, Oxford 1992, 248–9.
26 For Amsterdam and Dr Tulp, see Evenhuis, *Ook dat was Amsterdam*, 2, 76–7, see also Chapter 3 of this volume; for Jacob Viverius, see Grell, 'Conflicting Duties', 141 and 150.
27 For Emden, see Pettegree, *Emden and the Dutch Revolt*.
28 See *ibid.*, 36–7.
29 For Groningen, see F. Huisman, *Stadsbelang en standsbesef. Gezondheidszorg en medisch beroep in Groningen 1500–1730*, Rotterdam 1992, 163–71; see also Grell, 'The Religious Duty of Care', 259.
30 Huisman, *Stadsbelang en standsbesef*, 172–7.
31 See Chapter 4 of this volume.
32 For the close contacts between the Dutch Church in London and Antwerp, see O. P. Grell, *Exiles in Tudor and Stuart England*, Aldershot 1996, especially Chapters 1 and 5; for the regular assistance offered to the Reformed community by its sister church in London, see *Acta... van de Nederlandse Gemeente te Londen*, nos 685, 691, 698, 868, 1215, 1252, 1261, 1332, 2877, 2883; for contacts with Emden, see Pettegree, *Emden and the Dutch Revolt*.
33 For Assuerus Regemorter, see O. P. Grell, 'Merchants and Ministers: the foundations of international Calvinism', in A. Pettegree *et al.* (eds) *Calvinism in Europe 1540–1620*, Cambridge 1994, 261, 272; for Assuerus's statement in the London consistory, see *Acta... van de Nederlandse Gemeente te Londen*, 611.

34   For Radermacher's interest in medicine, see Grell, 'Merchants and Ministers', 272, note 74.

35   See Chapter 4 of this volume.

36   See Chapter 5 of this volume.

37   For the church orders for Hamburg and Lübeck, see E. Sehling (ed.) *Die evangelischen Kirchenordnungen des XVI Jahrhunderts*, V, Leipzig 1913, 334–68 and 488–540; see also F. P. Lane, 'Poverty and Poor Relief in the German Church Orders of Johann Bugenhagen 1485–1558', PhD thesis, Ohio State University 1973, 197–8 and 210–12.

38   For this, see Chapter 5 of this volume.

39   Sehling, *Kirchenordnungen*, 359.

40   *ibid.*, 360–61; see also Lane, 'Johann Bugenhagen', 214–5.

41   Lane, 'Johann Bugenhagen', 215.

42   For Andreas Hyperius, see R. Jütte, 'Andreas Hyperius (1511–64) und die Reform des Frühneuzeitlichen Armenwesens', *Archiv für Reformationsgeschichte*, 75, 1984, 113–38; for Hyperius's inspiration, see 121 in particular.

43   *ibid.*, 127–31.

44   See Chapter 5 of this volume.

45   See Chapter 6 of this volume.

46   We are grateful for this information to Mr Lars Bisgaard of the University of Odense, Denmark, who is presently engaged in writing a doctoral dissertation on the establishment of late medieval masses for the dead in Denmark.

47   For Riis's much more negative interpretation of these developments, see Chapter 6 of this volume. This rests on a different reading of the seminal article by T. Dahlerup, 'Den Sociale Forsorg og Reformationen i Danmark', *Historie. Jyske Samlinger*, Ny Rk. XIII, 1–2, 1979, 194–207, especially 203–7.

48   For Hamsfort, see P. R. Kruse, *Lægemiddelpriserne i Danmark indtil 1645. En undersøgelse af lovgivningen for fastsættelse af forbrugerprisen på lægemidler*, Copenhagen 1991, 51–9, especially 52.

49   For a general outline of this growing millenarianism in Europe, see F. A. Yates, *The Rosicrucian Enlightenment*, London 1986; for England in particular, see C. Webster, *The Great Instauration*.

50   See Chapter 7 of this volume.

51   See Chapters 3 and 7 of this volume.

52   See Chapter 7 of this volume.

53   Slack, *Poverty and Policy*, 173–82; and R. Jütte, *Poverty and Deviance in Early Modern Europe*, Cambridge 1994, 50–61.

54   See Chapter 7 of this volume.

55   See Chapter 8 of this volume.

56   See Chapter 8 of this volume.

57   For the Reformation in Danzig, see M. G. Müller, 'Protestant Confessionalisation in the Towns of Royal Prussia and the Practice of Religious Toleration in Poland-Lithuania', in O. P. Grell and B. Scribner (eds) *Tolerance and Intolerance in the European Reformation*, Cambridge 1996, 262–81, especially 270–80; see also Janusz Tazbir, 'Poland', in B. Scribner *et al.* (eds) *The Reformation in National Context*,

Cambridge 1994, 168–80; for the welfare reforms, see Chapter 9 of this volume.

58 For Italians in Antwerp, see P. Burke, 'Antwerpen, a Metropolis in Europe', in *Antwerp: Story of a Metropolis, 16th–17th Centuries*, ed. J. Van der Stock, Antwerp 1993, 49–57.

59 Another and probably more likely line of inspiration may well be the Italian Health Boards of Venice and Florence in particular, which had come into existence towards the end of the fifteenth century; see C. M. Cipolla, *Public Health and the Medical Profession in the Renaissance*, Cambridge 1976.

60 For Copenhagen, see Kruse, *Lægemiddelpriserne i Danmark*, 108–36. Initially the University of Groningen played a similar role *vis-à-vis* the city authorities and a *Collegium Medicum* was not founded until 1728; see Huisman, *Stadsbelang en standsbesef*, 201–23 and 398–403.

61 See Chapter 11 of this volume; for London's growth in this period, see P. Clark and P. Slack, *English Towns in Transition 1500–1700*, Oxford 1976, 62–83.

62 Pettegree, *Foreign Protestant Communities*, 31.

63 For Zwingli and poor relief, see L. P. Wandel, *Always Among Us: Images of the poor in Zwingli's Zurich*, Cambridge 1990; for Bishop Ridley's statement, see Chapter 11 of this volume.

64 Grell, *Dutch Calvinists*, 9, 34–5.

65 See Chapter 11 of this volume; for the Merchants Adventurers in Antwerp, see W. R. Baumann, *The Merchants Adventurers and the Continental Cloth Trade (1560s–1620s)*, New York 1990.

66 For this suggestion, see T. Sellin, *Pioneering in Penology: the Amsterdam Houses of Correction in the sixteenth and seventeenth centuries*, Philadelphia 1944, 20–2. For the economic upturn in the United Provinces and Holland in particular, see Israel, *Dutch Primacy in World Trade*, 38–79.

67 Sellin, *Pioneering in Penology*, 25–30. See also A. Hallema, *Geschiedenis van het gevangeniswezen hoofdzakelijk in Nederland*, The Hague 1958.

68 See A. T. van Deursen, *Plain Lives in a Golden Age: popular culture, religion and society in seventeenth-century Holland*, Cambridge 1991, 53–5.

69 See Chapter 11 of this volume.

70 For the two projects, see P. Slack, *Poverty & Policy in Tudor and Stuart England*, London 1988, 117–8; for William Marshall and Christopher St German, see DNB.

71 J. Guy, *Tudor England*, Oxford 1988, 122–3.

72 Slack, *Poverty and Policy*, 122, 125. See also P. Collinson, *The Elizabethan Puritan Movement*, rep. Oxford 1990.

73 Slack, *Poverty and Policy*, 124, 149; see also P. Collinson, *The Religion of Protestants: the church in English society 1559–1625*, Oxford 1982, 141–3.

74 Slack, *Poverty and Policy*, 125–6; for Sir Robert Wroth, see W. Hunt, *The Puritan Moment: the coming of revolution in an English county*, Cambridge MA 1983, 66, 80. Other Calvinists or Puritans on the committees were Francis Hastings, Nathaniel Bacon, Thomas Hoby and Anthony Cope.

75   See E. M. Leonard, *The Early History of English Poor Relief*, Cambridge 1900, and Slack, *Poverty and Policy*, 128–9.

76   For Scotland, see Chapter 10 of this volume.

77   Grell, *Dutch Calvinists*, 93–105; for the lists see Guildhall Library MS 7424 and 7497/8.

78   For the religious development, see Collinson, *Elizabethan Puritan Movement*.

79   Grell, *Dutch Calvinists*, 47–8; and Slack, *Poverty and Policy*, 154.

80   O. P. Grell, 'From Uniformity to Tolerance: the effects on the Dutch Church in London of reverse patterns in English church policy from 1634 to 1647', *Nederlands Archief voor Kerkgeschiedenis*, 66, 1986, 17–39, especially 39; and Chapter 11 of this volume. See also O. P. Grell, 'Godly Charity or Political Aid? Irish Protestants and international Calvinism, 1641–5', *Historical Journal*, 39, 3, 1996, 743–53.

81   For these pamphleteers, see Webster, *Great Instauration*, 288–300.

82   P. Chamberlen, *The Poore Mans Advocate, or, Englands Samaritan. Pouring Oyle and Wyne into the Wounds of the Nation. By making Present Provision for the Souldier and the Poor*, London 1649.

83   For Cook, see *Biographical Dictionary of British Radicals in the Seventeenth Century*, eds R. L. Greaves and R. Zaller, Brighton 1982, 1; and R. Brenner, *Merchants and Revolution: commercial change, political conflict, and London's overseas traders, 1550–1653*, Cambridge 1993, 572.

84   For medical education in Leiden, see O. P. Grell, 'The Attraction of Leiden University for English Students of Medicine and Theology, 1590–1642', in C. C. Barfoot and R. Todd (eds) *The Great Emporium: the Low Countries as a cultural crossroads in the Renaissance and the eighteenth century*, Amsterdam 1992, 83–104, especially 96–7. For William Petty's matriculation, see *Album Studiosorum Academiae Lugduno Batavae MDLXXV–MDCCLXXV*, The Hague 1875, under 26 May 1644.

85   W. Petty, *The Advice of W. P. to Mr. Samuel Hartlib for the Advancement of Some Particular Parts of Learning*, London 1648, 8–17. Petty's hospital is dealt with in detail by Webster, *Great Instauration*, 293–5.

86   Webster, *Great Instauration*, 295–300.

87   See T. C. Smout, *A History of the Scottish People 1560–1830*, London 1979, 84–5; and J. Goodare, 'Scotland', in B. Scribner *et al.* (eds) *The Reformation in National Context*, Cambridge 1994, 95–110.

88   See Chapter 10 of this volume, and Smout, *Scottish People*, 94–9.

89   See A. I. MacInnes, *Charles I and the Making of the Covenanting Movement 1625–1641*, Edinburgh 1991.

Chapter 2

The Protestant imperative of Christian care and neighbourly love

Ole Peter Grell

Three things spring to mind when examining the considerable output of research into poor relief and health care provison in early modern Europe which has appeared over the last twenty-five years. First, poor relief and poverty have preoccupied historians to the detriment of the related issue of health care provision. Thus medicine and health care have only been allowed the occasional guest appearance in the series of works on poor relief published in the wake of Natalie Zemon Davis' seminal article, 'Poor Relief, Humanism and Heresy', first printed in 1968.[1] Furthermore, as opposed to the considerable literature on the Mediterranean countries, separate works on health care provision and medicine have, apart from England, been lacking for Northern Europe, in particular the Baltic and North Sea region.[2] Second, this geographical lacuna of research into medicine and health care provision in Northern, Protestant Europe, is matched by a corresponding near paucity of research into poverty and poor relief, as demonstrated by most of the recent case studies which have focused exclusively on Western and Central Europe.[3]

Third, the significance of the Reformation for the reform of and changes in poor relief has come to be seen as negligible. Today it has become generally accepted among historians that neither Catholicism nor Protestantism influenced the developments of the characteristic features of early modern poor relief re-organisation, such as the pooling of revenues and resources in a common fund, the 'common chest', and the centralisation of relief agencies.[4] Instead, these reforms are now seen as inspired by civic leaders and Christian humanists who were responding not to religious reforms, but to the economic and demographic changes of the period. This was incidentally the conclusion which Natalie Davis reached in 1968, and it has so far been supported by most of the leading scholars in this field, such as Brian Pullan, Paul Slack, Hugo Soly and Robert Jütte.[5] The result has been that religion is no longer seen as an important factor; and even if Natalie Davis admitted that there were differences between Catholic and Protestant welfare arrangements, she clearly considered them to be of a cosmetic rather than a constituent nature.[6] Undoubtedly, the removal of religion from this scenario can to some extent be seen as a healthy reaction to the confessionally biased historiography which had characterised this field until the 1960s, but that this conclusion was reached by predominantly social historians, influenced by the radical cultural climate of the late 1960s, when the impact of neo-Marxism and economic explanations was strong, can hardly surprise. However, the unquestioning acceptance of these views by most Reformation historians is surprising. Especially since this interpretation turns out to correspond broadly with that originally launched in the late nineteenth century by the two Catholic Church historians, Georg Ratzinger and Franz Ehrle.[7] That Otto Winkelmann's response to Ratzinger and Ehrle, in his studies on poor relief in Nuremberg, Kitzingen, Regensburg and Ypres, has now been forgotten is perhaps understandable, but that the more recent articles by Harold Grimm and Carter Lindberg have been largely ignored is less excusable, even if Grimm and Lindberg are primarily concerned with Luther's influence and theological rationale for encouraging changes in poor relief.[8]

Susan Brigden's recent book *London and the Reformation* offers an excellent example of how what I would term the socio-economic interpretation, namely that the initative for changes in poor relief came from civic government as a response to social and economic changes, has come to dominate this period's history. In spite of pointing to the significant creation of the five hospitals of St Bartholomew's, Christ's, St Thomas's, Bethlem and Bridewell as major charitable and Protestant initiatives in the reign of Edward VI, and emphasising that the 'increase in charitable giving coincided – exactly – with the advance of Protestantism', Brigden is still prepared to disregard her own evidence and to see the reforms as a consequence of an enormous rise in pauperism and interpret the change as a response to 'a social necessity'.[9] These are words which cannot but remind the reader of Pullan's claim that it was the omnipresence of disease, crime and crisis which caused territorial states and municipal governments to respond in similar ways to these urgent social problems.[10]

As will appear, I am of the opinion that it is time to undertake a revision and re-examination of this explanation of the transformation of early modern poor relief. I do not think that the last few decades of research by social historians have proved the case conclusively that the Reformation had little or no impact on the reforms of charity and poor relief which were introduced in many European countries. Consequently, I shall draw attention to what I consider to be the major flaws in this argument. Furthermore, I shall argue that the Reformation was of particular importance for the reforms in poor relief and health care provision which took place in Northern Europe in the sixteenth century.

Let me start with the general observation that in an age which was profoundly dominated and shaped by faith, I find it difficult to accept that religion should not have shaped the public and private approach to the way the poor and the sick should be treated.

One of the main arguments against the Reformation as having been the motivator, and Protestantism the prime mover, in the innovations in poor relief has been that many of the most important changes predate the Reformation. But the fact that examples can be found, such as that of Johannes Geiler von Kaysersberg (1445–1510), a cathedral preacher in Strasburg, who as early as 1498 had begun arguing that civil authorities should be responsible for the poor and provide them with work, education and relief, does not necessarily prove that Protestantism did not motivate or strongly influence the changes themselves. Neither does the fact that poor laws were issued and common chests established in some of the German cities years before the start of the Reformation, as for instance the Regensburg Poor Law Statutes of 1515 and the Württemberg common chest, envisaged in legislation drawn up towards the end of the fifteenth century,[11] mean that the Reformation did not decidedly shape and accelerate these changes. Similarly, no historian of the Reformation itself would try and explain away the role of Luther and other Protestants in bringing about this event, just because many of their theological points had already been made by Erasmus and other Christian humanists.

This leads directly to the peculiarly contradictory position of the leading advocates of what I term the socio-economic interpretation, namely their rejection of Protestantism and the Reformation as the instigator of reform in the social domain, while simultaneously accepting Christian humanism as an important inspiration behind the civic reforms of the period.[12] As recently pointed out by Euan Cameron, 'separating the humanist and Protestant input into the social control legislation of the early Reformation is a difficult and probably quite artificial task'.[13] Why have the Protestant reformers and their social reforms been considered of little or no importance, while Christian humanists such as Juan Luis Vives (1526) and Jean de Vauzelles (1532) and their proposals, have been emphasised as important? After all, their suggestions come chronologically later than those of Luther and his collaborators. Perhaps it has something to do with the fact that the case studies which have served to promote this argument have all been concerned with cities where humanism for political, religious and geographical reasons remained an important force, as in the case of Lyon (Davis), Venice (Pullan), Bruges and Ypres. However, to see these cities as good examples of Catholic cities introducing the same reforms as Protestant centres, and hence as proof that the Reformation and Protestantism were of little consequence for the social reforms which were thus instituted across Europe, strikes me as missing the point. It also ignores the crucial fact that all these cities, including Venice, contained substantial Protestant minorities for a considerable period, quite apart from influential groups of Catholic, Christian humanists.[14] Rather than undermining the case for the significance of Protestantism for the social reforms these examples seem to enhance it.

Furthermore, the socio-economic interpretation also attaches far too little importance to the contemporary criticism from mainstream Catholics of the reforms in Ypres and Lyon. Thus, the mendicant orders in Ypres attacked the magistracy's reform (1525) as tainted with heresy, while the Catholic theologians at the Sorbonne warned the city council not to forbid begging or to appropriate church property and income for their new scheme for poor relief. The Sorbonne professors warned that this 'would be the part not of good Catholics, but of impious heretics, Waldensians, Wycliffites or Lutherans'.[15] In Lyon the proposals by Jean de Vauzelles for new welfare schemes to be introduced by the city fathers were attacked by the Dominican Prior, Nicolas Morin, as 'pernicious to Catholic piety'.[16]

Even the most influential tract on the reform of poor relief by any of the Christian humanists, Juan Luis Vives's *De Subventione Pauperum* (On the Support of the Poor), published in Bruges in

1526, was attacked by prominent Catholics such as the Bishop of Tournai as being heretical and Lutheran.[17] These Christian humanist proposals for social reform and the practical schemes they are seen to have inspired in Ypres and Lyon were, in other words, considered by contemporary, mainstream Catholics to be heavily influenced by Luther and Protestantism!

Considering Vives's contacts with German scholars it is more than likely that he had been influenced by Luther's views on poor relief which had already been widely publicised in his treatise of 1520, *To the Christian Nobility of the German Nation*. Vives may also have received information on the new poor relief schemes in Germany, as for instance that in Nuremberg (1522), from his friend, the Protestant preacher in Strasburg, Caspar Hedio, who later, in 1532, translated Vives's treatise into German.[18] Perhaps too much has been made of the originality and influence of Vives's tract on early modern poor relief. It certainly carried little weight in Northern Europe where the influence of Luther and his colleague and collaborator Johannes Bugenhagen became paramount. Vives's influence may well have been limited even in the Netherlands, where he resided. When, in 1526, he dedicated his tract *De Subventione Pauperum* to the magistracy of his home town, Bruges, the city's social reforms were already in place and the reforms in nearby Ypres had taken place the previous year.[19]

The fact that some of the poor relief reforms which took place in German cities, such as that of Nuremberg in 1522, were introduced well before the publication of Vives's treatise, has not stopped advocates of the socio-economic thesis from seeing them as inspired solely by Christian humanism. Considering Luther's close contacts with the civic leadership in Nuremberg from as early as 1518, in particular with Lazarus Spengler, this is difficult to accept. Especially since the Protestant motivation behind the new poor relief scheme in Nuremberg is clearly stated in its preamble:

> Faith and love, as Christ says in Matthew 22, are the two pillars of Christian existence, wherein are included all God's command-ments and on which all laws and the prophets depend. To love Christ and to depend on him alone, and to love my neighbour, as I believe Christ has taught me, that is the only true way to be godly and saved, and nothing else.[20]

Finally, the discrepancy in the chronology of the reforms in poor relief and health care provision between Protestant and Catholic

countries and cities seems to have received little attention. Even if
we accept that Christian humanism inspired Protestants, as well as
Catholics, the speed was faster and the changes far more radical in
Protestant areas, as can be seen from the Wittenberg Church Order
of 1522, the Nuremberg Poor Ordinance of 1522, and those of
Leisnig (1523), Kitzingen (1523) and Regensburg (1523), than
within Catholic areas, where the first ordinance, as far as I can see,
was that of Ypres (1525).[21] A similar discrepancy is apparent when
we examine who placed a renewed and enhanced emphasis on
discriminatory alms-giving and the prohibition of begging, aspects
which increasingly came to characterise post-Reformation charity.
With a couple of exceptions they were either Protestants or
Christian humanists, and more importantly, the few Catholic
exceptions consist of Counter-Reformation theologians such as
Ignatius Loyola and Miguel de Giginta, whose 'reformed Catholicism had incorporated many of the welfare policies originally
advocated by humanists and Protestants'.[22] This is also confirmed
by the examples provided by Pullan in an article from 1976. The
advocates of some form of discriminatory poor relief mentioned here
are all post-Tridentine theologians, such as Vincent de Paul.

Pullan has remained a strong advocate of the socio-economic
model, but he has emphasised that even within post-Tridentine
Catholicism, which saw the introduction of some differentiation
between the deserving and the undeserving poor, the Catholic focus
remained on the almsgiver and not on the receiver. Similarly, the
physical aid and assistance still came second to the main priority,
namely the salvation of the souls of both donor and receiver.

It is also noteworthy that Pullan, pointing to early modern
Catholic poor relief as a mixture of traditional and post-Tridentine
initiatives, draws attention to the prominent role of the Observant
Franciscans in creating the cheap loan facilities for the poor, the
Monte di Pieta, which achieved such importance in Italy in the
sixteenth century, and in the Italian hospital reforms which
preceded the Reformation by seventy years. Likewise Pullan
underlines the importance for Catholic charity of the re-invigoration
of the confraternities, especially in Southern Europe.[23] But these
were exactly the organisations which in their unreconstituted form
in Northern Europe became the target for some of the most
venomous attacks by the Protestant reformers, starting with Luther's
treatise from 1519, *The Blessed Sacrament of the Holy and the True Body
of Christ, and the Brotherhoods*. Apart from constituting the main

challenge to the Protestant reformers in most towns and cities, not least because of their vernacular preaching, it should not be forgotten that the mendicant orders were primarily geared to saving souls, and only as a consequence of that were they concerned with practical charity. In spite of the Observant movement which after all enhanced the traditional Catholic position, that a truly evangelical life was one led in voluntary poverty after the example of Christ, the emphasis continued to be on the beneficence to lay Christians of such ecclesiastical orders. Looking at the impressive Franciscan and Dominican monastic buildings in the modest towns and cities of early modern Northern Europe which have survived, we are reminded that it was mainly the monks and friars who benefited from the Observant movement, primarily because of their spiritual services, such as prayers, vigils and masses for the dead. Considering that the mendicant orders were prevented from owning property and real estate, the monetary donations they received must have been enormous. Luther had already pointed this out in 1520, when he noted that if his suggestion for the abolition of begging was introduced there were those who would claim that 'the poor would not be so well provided for, that fewer great stone houses and monasteries would be built, and fewer so well furnished'. He added that he could 'well believe all this, but none of it is necessary'.[24] Clearly, when competing with these voluntary, ecclesiastical poor for public charity the prospects for the lay, involuntary poor must have been depressing.[25] The religious confraternities, which occupied a peculiar position somewhere between the lay and ecclesiastical sphere, were also, in spite of their charity, particularly towards their own members, primarily concerned with the afterlife. They are probably best described as 'friendly societies where premiums were paid in good works and the rewards matured in eternal life'.[26] As such they received fierce criticism in Luther's treatise *To the Christian Nobility of the German Nation*:

> Compared with the true brotherhood in Christ those brotherhoods are like a penny to a gulden. But if there were a brotherhood which raised money to feed the poor or to help the needy, that would be a good idea. It would find its indulgences and merits in heaven. But today nothing comes of these groups except gluttony and drunkenness.[27]

Even if the mendicant orders and the confraternities did indeed justify their existence with the doctrine of good works, whereby a person's meritorious actions, channelled through the church, contributed to their own salvation, historians have shown an unfortunate preoccupation with this doctrine. Thus, I agree with Pullan, that the scholarly concentration on the doctrine of good works has been 'not so much incorrect as unduly narrow'.[28] Admittedly, the emphasis on faith and grace by the Protestant reformers made the doctrine of good works look like yet another invention by Rome, but what mattered just as much in this context was Luther's definition of the church as the 'Priesthood of all believers'. This was a crucial point, denying that priestly orders made someone a superior Christian and that the church possessed sole or privileged access to holiness and God.[29] It served to hand the church back to the laity by redefining it as a Christian community with no qualitative difference between clergy and laity. The emphasis shifted away from celibacy towards marriage, and the godly, Protestant family became the cornerstone of the Christian community.[30] This emphasis on the family was prominent in most Protestant church orders, specifically in the sections dealing with those officials who were to be put in charge of the new schemes for poor relief. In the Braunschweig Order of 1528 it was pointed out that prospective deacons had to be chosen from among upright family men who were known to provide well for their own children and households. Clearly for the reformers charity began at home and unless already demonstrated within the narrow confines of family and household, could not be expected to be extended by prospective deacons to the community at large.[31]

For Protestants charity became a Christian obligation within the civic, Christian Commonwealth. 'You shall love your neighbour as yourself' became the Protestant rationale for charity, as a consequence of and proof of faith and grace.[32] Thus the role of the voluntary poor such as the mendicant orders was obsolete if not downright negative. Solely by removing them and the confraternities Protestantism cannot but have improved the chances of the impoverished sections of the laity.

A number of historians have correctly emphasised that the reward motive in connection with good works continued to play a part in Protestant charity, but it did so with a significant difference.[33] Where Catholic charity was performed with the certainty of reward in the afterlife – being claims already underwritten by the church – Protestant donors had no such guarantees, and their hope of reward could never be more than a pious hope, which found continuous expression in a religious context where clerical middlemen no longer existed to ease the Christian individual's troubled journey towards salvation.

Because Protestant charity became solely a civil obligation towards the Christian Commonwealth, it focused on the living, and on the present as opposed to the hereafter. It treated the poor as subjects, as unfortunate Christian brethren and sisters who had justifiable expectations of assistance from their Christian community, which in turn had the right to make its own demands on its poor. This, as we have seen, differed starkly from the rationale of Catholic charity which continued to be preoccupied with the salvation of the donor's soul in particular, and to treat the poor as objects, even after the post-Tridentine reforms.

Without the Reformation the centralisation and increased accountability of poor relief which took place in the sixteenth- and seventeenth centuries would have been unimaginable.[34] That the unintended consequence of the Reformation for European poor relief took the reforms further than the laicisation which the reformers intended, to the secularisation they probably never imagined, is best explained by the failure to permanently Protestantise society.

The optimism which characterised the early reformers during the first years of the Reformation quickly evaporated. It proved much harder to convert the majority of the people than they had expected, even where the Reformation was strongly backed by government. Similarly, the reformers' high hopes for the reforms of charity and poor relief met with some early disappointments, as can be seen from Luther's letter to Spalatin where he pointed out that the reforms in Leisnig (1523) had not been as successful as he had hoped.[35] But these examples do not necessarily mean that the Reformation and the reforms of poor relief failed, only that the reformers' expectations were too great. In the short term, the changes introduced by the reformers undoubtedly caused confusion and bewilderment and may well, as in the case of England, have reduced existing sources of charity in the short term.[36] But even that is far from definite. First, we do not know how many of the medieval resources for charity were actually used directly to assist the involuntary poor: most of them may well have been spent on purely ecclesiastical purposes. Second, in Northern Europe the post-Reformation sources concerning charity differ significantly from the medieval ones – no longer are we dealing primarily with wills and letters of donations: instead we have administrative sources, letters of complaints, drafts for reforms, etc. This is a source material which by its nature focuses on shortcomings and failures, as opposed to the medieval material which records the positive events.[37]

As already mentioned, I think it is a meaningless enterprise to try to separate Christian humanist ideas for the reform of poor relief from similar Protestant plans. But where the Christian humanists wrote treatises about the reform of charity, and were only occasionally, like De Vauzelles in Lyon, involved in the practical reforms, the Protestant reformers of Northern Europe incorporated their plans for changes in health care and poor relief into their new church orders, which were directly concerned with practical reforms on the ground. The reformers were not satisfied with tinkering with one aspect of society only. Instead, they considered their social reforms to be a necessary and important dimension of the overall Reformation of church and society.[38] What had been a good option for Christian humanists became an obligation for good Protestants.

The single most influential Protestant reformer of poor relief and health care provision in Northern Europe was undoubtedly, Luther's friend and collaborator, Johannes Bugenhagen. Bugenhagen, born into a burgher family in the small town of Wollin in Pomerania in 1485, came to dominate the reforms from 1526 onwards. Where Luther started, Bugenhagen followed. His influence in the region we are concerned with is demonstrated not only by the six church orders he helped draw up, starting with Braunschweig in 1528, Hamburg in 1529, Lübeck in 1531, Pomerania 1535, Denmark in 1537-9, and Schleswig-Holstein in 1542; but also by his public letters to the people of England and Livonia, in which he defended Lutheranism.[39]

Bugenhagen's contributions to the social reforms are generally considered to have been insubstantial and mainly pertaining to the administration of poor relief, with one exception: the division of the common chest into two chests, one exclusively for the poor, the other for salaries of ministers and teachers and expenses for the upkeep of churches.[40] This was done in order to make it easier for the Protestant preachers to exhort their congregations to give liberally to the poor without being accused of acting out of self-interest, secretly trying to increase their salaries.[41] Where this division was not introduced, as in Denmark and Schleswig-Holstein, the church orders emphasised that the ministers could still exhort their congregations with a 'good conscience and without suspicion of avariciousness' since they were not to benefit from such charity.[42]

With regard to the reform of poor relief, its detailed administration, the definition of the deserving and undeserving poor, and antagonism towards begging, Bugenhagen added little to what Luther and others had already advocated. Instead, his contribution was in the area which we label health care provision. In this connection it is worth remembering that Luther and his collaborators had given little attention to these issues in either the Wittenberg *Beutelordnung* of 1521, the Wittenberg Church Order of 1522 or the Ordinance for a Common Chest for Leisnig in 1523. Thus, the issue was just mentioned briefly in the Leisnig Ordinance where it was stated that assistance should be given to the poor, infirm and aged 'out of Christian love, to the honor and praise of God, so that their lives and health may be preserved from further deterioration, enfeeblement, and foreshortening through lack of shelter, clothing, nourishment and care'.[43]

For Bugenhagen health care provision became as essential a part of a proper Protestant church order as the reform of poor relief had originally been for Luther. The attention these issues received in Bugenhagen's church orders centred around four main points: baptism, midwifery, nursing and hospitals. Even if there may have been a considerable local input in these orders, Bugenhagen's awareness of and emphasis on these matters appears to have increased over time. Let me begin by taking a closer look at baptism, which may at first glance seem the least obvious point for inclusion here.

BAPTISM

The Protestant reformers in their ambition to demolish the sacramental power held by the medieval Catholic Church, decided to retain only two of the sacraments, the eucharist and baptism, and then only in a strongly modified form.[44] Apart from the changed importance attached to baptism, it was no longer considered absolutely necessary for salvation, and unbaptised children were no longer consigned to limbo. The reformers also cleansed the ceremony of what they considered unnecessary and superstitious practices. Out went the annointment with chrism (consecrated balsam and oil), the sign of the cross with holy water, the use of the chrisom (a white cloth bound around the child's head, in which it should be buried if it died in infancy), the lighting of candles, etc.[45] What remained was the cleansing and salvation of the soul through the 'living water', as mentioned in the Bible. Referring to Ephesians 5:25ff the Braunschweig Order states: 'From these words you hear that Christ himself with the Holy Ghost baptises you and washes away your sins in the baptism with water, making you an eternal child of God's'.[46] Bugenhagen emphasised this even more strongly in the Lübeck Church Order of 1531. Writing about the 'glorious baptism with water' Bugenhagen stated that it was 'a bath of rebirth and renewal by the Holy Ghost' which washes away all sins.[47] This stress on the spiritual cleansing of the baptised child shifted the focus away from the sacrament (as absolutely necessary for salvation) and its significance for the hereafter, towards the living child. This is further amplified by Bugenhagen's Church Orders for Hamburg and Denmark.

In some parts of Northern Europe, most likely as a consequence of the cold climate but probably also encouraged by the evangelical movement, it had become common practice to have children baptised swaddled as opposed to naked, with water poured only over their heads.[48] As far as I can see, this practice was first recorded in the new Protestant Church Order for the territory of Hadeln near Bremen which was issued in 1526. It stated that children should be baptised by having water scooped over their head three times and added: 'In winter the sexton shall heat the water in a dish and put that in the font. Because baptism is for healing not harming'.[49] Bugenhagen evidently accepted this practice, as can be seen from his Church Order for Hamburg (1529):

> Since the practice only to baptise with water over the head may in time be abandoned by us, and the common practice used all over Germany, in other countries and by our neighbours, may be introduced here, and in order that imprudent people through hasty changes should not commit errors, like those who consider baptism with water on the head only to be invalid, which it is not, as already said: it is a proper baptism with water in the name of the Trinity, as commanded by Christ.

The common German practice which Bugenhagen referred to was to baptise the child naked or loosely dressed, the minister scooping or pouring water from the font with his right hand over the back and head of the child three times. However, in winter when this might prove dangerous to the child, the sexton should be instructed to heat the water as suggested in the Hadeln Order.[50]

A slightly different description can be found in the Danish Church Order of 1539. Here it is stated that children should be uncovered, but only that water should be scooped or poured over them three times, without specifying whether or not it should be applied to the head solely. However, it states that the guiding principle was to be the health of the children. If at risk from bad weather or disease the children should remain swaddled, because 'it was children's welfare not their harm which was sought through baptism'.[51] Bugenhagen's main collaborator in the Danish Church Order, the first Protestant Bishop of Zealand, Peder Palladius,[52] underlined the Protestant concern for the health aspect in connection with baptism in a special section of his *Visitation-Book* entitled 'About the font in particular':

> The font shall always remain dry and clean without water until a Danish child comes to church to be baptised, then the parish clerk or the sexton shall pour a bucket or two of water in the font, in order to prevent the water from being dirty and full of woodlice and similar filth (if you will excuse me) so that you would be loathe to dip a finger in it, let alone baptise a child in it, but there shall always be clean and clear water in it, like our Lord Jesus was baptised in clean and clear, running water from the river Jordan.

Palladius continued by stressing that in winter water should be warmed for this purpose, 'because baptism has been given our children for the salvation of their souls not for any harm or destruction of their bodies'.[53]

Thus for Protestants the significance attached to baptism lessened. No longer was it considered absolutely necessary for salvation and the afterlife. Instead, the emphasis shifted away from the dead rite towards the living receiver, as prominently demonstrated in the growing concern for the health of the child.

MIDWIFERY

As was the case with the reforms of poor relief, the first attempts to regulate midwifery had already started in some German cities towards the end of the fifteenth century. For doctrinal reasons alone it became important for Protestants to supervise midwives, not least because of their central role in emergency baptisms. Bugenhagen accordingly included separate sections about midwives in his church orders. In the Braunschweig Church Order Bugenhagen emphasised that the midwives were to be educated and visited by the local minister or superintendent in order to make sure that they were of sound doctrine, while a group of 'honourable and wise women' appointed by the magistracy should make sure that only upright and honest women were licensed as midwives. Apart from these doctrinal and moral concerns, however, the Braunschweig Order is primarily concerned with providing a reasonable and reliable service for the Christian community in Braunschweig. It wanted to remedy the shortage of qualified midwives which affected poorer families in particular. It stated that it was a Christian obligation for the community to provide enough, qualified, midwives, supported by the common chest, covering all sectors of the town. Poor women should enjoy their services free of charge while women who were not destitute should continue to pay.[54] Most of this was repeated in the Danish Church Order of 1539: it was a Protestant obligation to make sure that 'honest and pious' midwives were widely available to assist the rich as well as the poor, but nothing was said about how this was to be achieved or financed.[55] In his *Visitation-Book*, Bishop Peder Palladius encouraged women to pay good midwives generously, and town councils to exempt them from all taxes. Furthermore, Palladius advocated the practice already known from Germany whereby 'honourable women' exercised control over the appointment of midwives. This system has been interpreted as a municipal way of controlling a 'profession' which was predominantly recruited from the lower classes.[56] This may have been the intention in some German towns, but for the first Protestant Bishop of Zealand the motivation would appear to have been the ambition to secure the best possible care for pregnant women:

> And the eldest and most excellent Danish women in the parishes or in the town should inquire whether or not she (the midwife) is good at her office, before she is allowed to attend any Danish women, otherwise everything is lost; the child who is dead, is dead, he who is ruined, is ruined, the goose who has lost its head, does not gaggle, as the saying goes.
>
> Who wants to have his child killed, who wants his wife ruined, how many are those who have been destroyed by evil and ungodly midwives? Accordingly, it is of the utmost importance,

for men as well as women, that the midwife is a good, learned and pious woman, because no-one wants to see any of his nearest ruined.[57]

This increased concern with the physical care of mother and child was not unique to Palladius and Denmark, but was a characteristic element of Protestant care. Still, it may be advisable to take the results of a recent study of midwifery in the seventeenth century in a small town in Germany with a mixed population of Catholics and Protestants which has revealed that the post-birth death rate of Catholic mothers and infants (attended by Catholic midwives) was much higher than that of Protestants (attended by Protestant midwifes) from the same social stratum, with some reservations.[58]

NURSING

A further example of Bugenhagen's deep concern with the obligation of the properly reformed Christian Commonwealth to provide care in the community, can be found in his attempts to establish some form of nursing service. In the Church Orders for Braunschweig and Hamburg a paragraph was inserted which specified that the ministers should keep a register of the names of all the women who were maintained in the hospital and of all those who received regular support from the common chest. These women were obliged to nurse the sick, except when they had small children of their own or sick members of their immediate family. It was underlined that these women were to be remunerated either from the common chest, if their patients were poor, or by the patients personally.

However, should any of these women refuse to undertake such duties they were to be excluded from the hospital and from regular pay-outs from the common chest. In this Protestant version of the Christian Commonwealth the poor not only had a rightful claim on assistance from the local community, but also an obligation to contribute to society.[59]

Similarly, in his advice for the administration of the common chest in the Church Order for Pomerania (1535), Bugenhagen emphasized that the deacons should never spend all the money in the chest, but hold something in reserve for the poor who fell sick suddenly or who were about to give birth.[60] Bishop Peder Palladius emphasised this Protestant obligation to care for the sick in a paragraph in his *Visitation-Book* where he rejected the Catholic practice of pilgrimages to shrines as an ungodly activity:

> But holiness, that is to visit God's true sanctuary, God's living temple, in particular on holidays, who is your neighbour, Iacob, Søffren, Anne, who lie on their sickbeds, being the living flesh and blood, who lie smarting and aching,... [61]

HOSPITALS

Initially Bugenhagen's church orders appear to have concentrated exclusively on the need to establish plague hospitals. This is hardly surprising since Johannes Bugenhagen had recent and personal experience of a serious epidemic in which, among others, his sister had died. Together with Luther, Bugenhagen had remained in Wittenberg during 1527 when plague raged in the city for six months, in order to minister to his congregation and to lecture to his students. [62]

In Braunschweig the plague hospital was to be placed outside the city, while in Hamburg it was to constitute a separate part of a new, large hospital, but in all cases it was to have a number of separate chambers for the plague-stricken to make sure they did not infect each other. These hospitals were to be supplied with a salaried nursing staff in times of plague. The common chest was also to pay for food, beds, medicine and other necessities for the patients. The Braunschweig Order indicated that when the patients' families or masters did not meet the expenses incurred, the costs should be borne by the common chest. It emphasised that only heathens would incarcerate plague victims without providing for their physical needs, underlining that their isolation also served to protect the healthy. [63] However, in the Hamburg Order, issued the following year, it had become a 'Christian obligation' for the victims' masters and families to pay the costs in order not to put unnecessary strain on the public purse. [64]

Considering that syphilis or pox, which first appeared in Europe in 1495, seems to have spread with particular speed in the decade leading up to 1520, [65] it is understandable that it should receive special attention in some of Bugenhagen's church orders. The need for a separate pox hospital is first mentioned in the Church Order for Lübeck issued in 1531. [66] Pox also featured eight years later in the Danish Church Order. Concerning hospitals, the Danish Order specified that the sick should be isolated in separate rooms in the hospital, according to their type of disease, in order to prevent diseases from spreading, especially in cases which were feared to be of an epidemic nature. Pox, which was here considered a curable disease, was given a special mention. The Order emphasised that the town physicians should do their utmost to cure syphilitics and other sick, against payment, 'in order that the poor are not only kept alive, but are helped to improve their health as much as possible'.[67]

Syphilis was evidently of great concern in Northern Europe in the 1520s and 30s. When, in 1528, the Danish Christian humanist and Carmelite friar, Paulus Helie, was asked for advice about the foundation of a new hospital by one of the burgomasters of Copenhagen, Niels Stemp, he suggested not only that a pox hospital be established in the city, but in all the other major Danish towns.[68] Likewise, when Peder Palladius identified the deserving poor for his readers, he wrote:

> But if you want to see who receive your charity, then, when you are in Copenhagen on some other business, go to the hospital of the Holy Spirit, which is in the centre, where you will find the door open and walk along one side of the hospital and then the other and you will see how many poor alms-receivers lie in these beds from all over Zealand, whose noses, eyes and mouths have been eaten away by the pox, and whose arms and legs have rotted away through cancer and pain and still rot by worms and maggots, none of whom will ever be cured.[69]

The horror of such a visit was intended to remind the visitor of his own good and, importantly, undeserved fortune, thus encouraging him to show greater charity towards his less fortunate neighbours.

Undoubtedly, there were several aspects of these hospital reforms which had already been introduced elsewhere well before the Reformation, both in Italy and southern Germany. Thus Bugenhagen would have found plenty of support from Christian humanists, such as Paulus Helie for his ambition to forbid wealthy pensioners buying themselves old-age care in the hospitals.[70] Similarly little or nothing would have separated the Protestant reformers from Christian humanists concerning the administration of hospitals. Where funds proved insufficient, despite attempts to retain donations, previously given to the Catholic Church, for the new, Protestant establishments, reformers as well as humanists agreed that lay government had an obligation to step in.[71]

Let me conclude by emphasising that by seeking to re-insert the Reformation into the story about early modern innovations in poor relief and health care provision, I am not arguing that Protestantism alone brought about these changes, or that social and economic factors were of little or no consequence, but only that the Reformation was responsible for the speed and to some extent for the nature of these changes. My arguments have focused on the significance of the early Lutheran Reformation in bringing about these changes, but I am convinced that a similar case could be argued for Calvinism and Reformed Protestantism when and where it made an impact, as has recently been forcefully shown in the case of the English town of Dorchester in the early seventeenth century by David Underdown.[72]

In other words what concerns me here is not the early Reformation *per se* in a chronological sense, but early rather in a generational sense. Thus it is of little consequence whether the Reformation was Lutheran or Reformed in character, or if it took place in the early sixteenth century or a century later, but whether the reforms were driven by a strong sense of religious urgency and a commitment towards establishing a new Christian Commonwealth. This often had a strong millenarian tinge which might occasionally serve to revive a Protestant urge for reform which was seldom sustainable for more than a generation.

Thus it was Protestant reformers such as Johannes Bugenhagen who gave much needed urgency and theological justification to these reforms. Built into their reformation of church and state was the ambition to create a Christian Commonwealth which possessed the proper institutions for providing for the sick and the poor. For them, this consisted of a reciprocal arrangement whereby the Christian community had an obligation to look after its destitute members with the aim of helping them once more to become valuable members of society, while the poor, on the other hand, were obliged to undertake some form of service to the community, if need be, and, if they were not already fully committed looking after their own, destitute families. By nature, such arrangements imposed a degree of social control on the poorer members of society. Perhaps historians of the post-Foucault era have made too much of the control side of these reforms and forgotten the care aspect, which, after all, was the motivation which caused so many of the Protestant reformers to emphasise the importance of reforms to poor relief and health care provision in their church orders.

NOTES

1 N. Z. Davis, 'Poor Relief, Humanism and Heresy' republished in N. Z. Davis, *Society and Culture in Early Modern France*, Stanford 1975, 17–64.

2 See the recent survey by R. Jütte, *Poverty and Deviance in Early Modern Europe*, Cambridge 1994. For Scandinavia, see the recent volume edited by T. Riis, which, however, concentrates on the eighteenth century, *Aspects of Poverty in Early Modern Europe III. La Pauvreté dans les Pays Nordiques 1500–1800*, Odense 1990.

3 R. Jütte, *Poverty and Deviance in Early Modern Europe*, 1.

4 See R. W. Scribner, 'Politics and Institutionalisation of Reform in Germany', in G. R. Elton (ed.) *The Reformation 1520–59, The New Cambridge Modern History*, vol. 2, 2nd ed., Cambridge 1990, 177–8.

5 B. Pullan, *Rich and Poor in Renaissance Venice*, Oxford 1971; C. Lis and H. Soly (eds) *Poverty and Capitalism in Pre-Industrial Europe*, Hassocks, Sussex, 1979; P. Slack, *Poverty and Policy in Tudor and Stuart England*, London 1988; R. Jütte, *Poverty and Deviance in Early Modern Europe*, Cambridge 1994.

6 N. Z. Davis, 'Poor Relief', 60.

7 G. Ratzinger, *Geschichte der Kirchlichen Armenplege*, Freiburg 1868–84; and F. Ehrle, *Beiträge zur Geschichte und Reform der Armenplege*, Freiburg 1881.

8 O. Winkelmann, 'Die Armenordnung von Nürnberg (1522), Kitzingen (1523), Regensburg (1523) und Ypern (1525)', I and II, *ARG* (Archiv für Reformationsgeschichte), 10 (1913), 242–80, and *ARG*, 11 (1914), 1–18; O. Winkelmann, 'Über die ältesten Armenordnungen der Reformationszeit (1521–25)', *Historisches Vierteljahrsschrift*, XVII (1914), 187–228, 361–400; H. J. Grimm, 'Luther's Contributions to Sixteenth-Century Organization of Poor Relief', *ARG*, 61 (1970), 222–34; C. Lindberg, ' "There Should Be No Beggars Among Christians": Karlstadt, Luther, and the origins of Protestant poor relief', *Church History*, 46 (1977) no. 3, 313–34.

9 S. Brigden, *London and the Reformation*, Oxford 1989, 477, 481–2.

10 Pullan, *Rich and Poor*, 223–4 and 638.

11 Scribner, 'Politics', 178. See also R. W. Scribner, 'Paradigms of Urban Reform', in L. Grane and K. Hørby (eds) *Die Dänische Reformation vor ihrem Internationalen Hintergrund*, Göttingen 1990, 125.

12 See Davis, 'Poor relief', 60; Slack, *Poverty and Policy*, 9; Jütte, *Poverty*, 106.

13 Cameron, *European Reformation*, 259.

14 For Lyon, see N. Z. Davis, 'Strikes and Salvation at Lyon', in N. Z. Davis, *Society and Culture*, 1–16; for Venice, see E. Cameron, 'Italy', in A. Pettegree (ed.) *The Early Reformation in Europe*, Cambridge 1992, 188–214, especially 198 and 204–5. For Bruges and Ypres, see J. Briels, *Zuid-Nederlanders in de Republiek 1572–1630*, Danthe, Sint-Niklaas 1985, 35–6, 45–8.

15 Grimm, 'Luther's Contributions', 232; the statement of the theologians at the Sorbonne is cited by Davis in 'Poor relief', 17.

16   Cited in Davis, 'Poor Relief', 17.
17   *ibid.*
18   Grimm, 'Luther's Contributions', 232.
19   Jütte, *Poverty*, 112–13; see also Cameron, *The European Reformation*, 259.
20   The Nuremberg poor relief order of 1522 is published in Winkelmann, 'Armenordnung', 258–80 (my translation).
21   Luther personally wrote the introduction to the Ordinance for Leisnig; see E. Sehling (ed.) *Die evangelischen Kirchenordnungen des XVI. Jahrhunderts*, vol. 1, part 1, Leipzig 1902, 596–604. The Protestant inspiration for the Ordinances for Kitzingen and Regensburg are as pronounced as in that already quoted from Nuremberg, whereas that for Ypres lacks a similar justification, see Winkelmann, 'Armenordnungen', *ARG*, 11 (1914), 1–2, 8–9, 13–14.
22   See Figure 10 in Jütte, *Poverty*, 101; Jütte has listed De Vauzelles and Vives as Catholic theologians there, whereas he refers to them as Christian humanists elsewhere in this book.
23   B. Pullan, 'Catholics and the Poor in Early Modern Europe', *Transactions of the Royal Historical Society*, 5th series, 26 (1976), especially 27–30.
24   H. T. Lehmann (ed.) *Luther's Works*, 44, Philadelphia 1961, 188
25   For the Observant movement, see Cameron, *The European Reformation*, 40–3. In this connection it is noteworthy that Dutch towns and cities saw their reformation in the 1570s as an opportunity to eliminate competing institutions of poor relief such as the monastic orders, the guilds and the confraternities, who often possessed much greater financial resources than the municipal poor masters; see A. Pettegree, 'The Calvinist Church in Holland, 1572–90', in A Pettegree *et al.* (eds) *Calvinism in Europe 1540–1620*, Cambridge 1994, 170. Clearly the success of the Christian humanists had been extremely limited in what became the United Provinces.
26   I have borrowed this expression from Pullan, 'Catholics and the Poor', 30.
27   Cited in Lindberg, 'There Should be No Beggars', 317. See *Luther's Works*, 44, 193.
28   Pullan, 'Catholics and the Poor', for quotation, see 34.
29   For an excellent discussion of the implications of the 'Priesthood of all believers', see Cameron, *The European Reformation*, 148–51.
30   For this, see S. Ozment, *When Fathers Ruled: family life in Reformation Europe*, Cambridge MA 1983; see also P. Collinson, *The Birthpangs of Protestant England: religious and cultural change in the sixteenth and seventeenth centuries*, London 1992, 60–93.
31   See Sehling, *Kirchenordnungen*, VI, part 1, 449.
32   *Matt.* 22.39; *Mark* 12.31.
33   See, for instance, Pullan, 'Catholics and the Poor', 21; Brigden, *London*, 482.
34   See Jütte, *Poverty*, 108.
35   *ibid.*, 107.

36 J. J. Scarisbrick, *The Reformation and the English People*, Oxford 1984, Chapter 2.

37 See the excellent article by T. Dahlerup, 'Den sociale forsorg og reformationen i Danmark', *Historie*, New Series, 13, nos. 1–2 (1979), 194–207.

38 Apart from the Church Orders which tended to be the work of Bugenhagen, it has been estimated that Luther influenced more than twenty-five poor ordinances in Germany between 1522–30, see Jütte, *Poverty*, 107; see also Grimm, 'Luther's Contributions'.

39 For Bugenhagen, see H.-G. Leder, 'Johannes Bugenhagen Pomeranus–Leben und Wirken', in H.-G. Leder (ed.) *Johannes Bugenhagen. Gestalt und Wirkung*, Berlin 1985, 8–37; for the Church Orders, see 24–9. For the letter to England, *Epistola ad Anglos*, (1525), see Brigden, *London*, 116. This letter was translated into English and published, *A Compendius Letter which Jhon Pomerane... - sent to the faythfull christen congregation in Engelande*, London 1536; see also the published response by Sir Thomas More, *A Reply to Bugenhagens Epistola ad Anglos*, London 1536.

40 See Jütte, *Poverty*, 107–8, and F. P. Lane, 'Poverty and Poor Relief in the German Church Orders of Johann Bugenhagen 1485–1558', PhD thesis, Ohio State University 1973. see also Chapter 5 of this volume.

41 This argument is first introduced into the Braunschweig Order (1528), see Sehling, *Kirchenordnungen*, VI, part 1, Tübingen 1955, 451; for Lübeck (1529), see Sehling, *Kirchenordnungen*, V, Leipzig 1913, 532.

42 For the Danish Church Order of 1539, see H. F. Rørdam (ed.) *Danske Kirkelove*, 1, Copenhagen 1881, 40–133; for this issue, see 113.

43 Sehling, *Kirchenordnungen*, I, part 1, 602; the translation is from H. T. Lehmann (ed.) *Luther's Works*, 45, Philadelphia 1962, 189. See also Grimm, 'Luther's Contributions', 226–8 and Lindberg, 'There Should be No Beggars', 327.

44 For Protestantism and the sacraments, see Cameron, *The European Reformation*, 156–67.

45 See K. Thomas, *Religion and the Decline of Magic*, Harmondsworth 1985, 40–1, and 63–4.

46 Sehling, *Kirchenordnungen*, VI, part 1, 355.

47 *ibid.*, V, 353.

48 Affusion (pouring water over the child), as opposed to immersion and submersion, as a form of baptism within the Catholic Church does not appear to have come into use until the later Middle Ages; see *The Oxford Dictionary of the Christian Church*, ed. F. L. Cross, Oxford 1978.

49 Sehling, *Kirchenordnungen*, V, 461.

50 *ibid.*, 511.

51 Rørdam, *Danske Kirkelove*, 1, 68. Swaddling seems to have been the custom in post-Reformation Denmark. This would explain the peculiar decision of the diocesan synod of Zealand in 1554: 'Children should be bare at baptism, in order to prevent people who practice witchcraft (veneficia) from trying to have wax models baptised in order to use them for witchcraft', see H. F, Rørdam, 'Forhandlinger

paa Roskilde Landemode 1554–59', *Kirkehistoriske Samlinger*, new series, 2, (1860–2), 450. This is also confirmed by the altar painting from Torslunde Church in Zealand from 1561 which shows the child swaddled (Nationalmuseet in Copenhagen).

52 For Peder Palladius, see M. Schwarz Lausten, 'The early Reformation in Denmark and Norway 1520–59', in O. P. Grell (ed.) *The Scandinavian Reformation: from evangelical movement to the institutionalisation of reform*, Cambridge 1995, 12–41.

53 *Peder Palladius' Danske Skrifter*, ed. L Jacobsen, V, Copenhagen 1925–6, 33–4.

54 Sehling, *Kirchenordnungen*, VI, part 1, 359–62, especially 359. For midwifery in this period, see M. E. Wiesner, 'The midwives of south Germany and the public/private dichotomy', in H. Marland (ed.) *The Art of Midwifery: The early modern midwives in Europe*, London 1993, 77–94

55 Rørdam, *Danske Kirkelove*, 1, 86–8.

56 See Wiesner, 'The midwives', 80–1.

57 *Peder Palladius' Skrifter*, V, 109 and 112. Palladius also appears to have been deeply concerned about the dangers of drunken midwives, see 112.

58 See M. Weisner, *Women and Gender in Early Modern Europe*, Cambridge 1993, 69. The discrepancy between the Catholic and Protestant post-birth death rate may be explained by the fact that Catholic midwives often baptised dead children on the parents' insistence, in the hope that these children might avoid limbo. Recent French research would indicate that around 20 per cent of the Catholic death rate may have been due to this practice (I should like to thank Professor E. A. Wrigley of Corpus Christi College, Cambridge, for drawing this to my attention). That it was a custom which was difficult to eradicate can be seen from the constant emphasis in Protestant church orders that midwives under no circumstances were allowed to baptise stillborn children.

59 Sehling, *Kirchenordnungen*, V, 508 and VI, part 1, 383.

60 *ibid.*, IV, Leipzig 1911, 337.

61 *Peder Palladius' Skrifter*, V, 132. For Peder Palladius' general attitude to charity, see M. Schwarz Lausten, *Biskop Peder Palladius og Kirken 1537–60*, Copenhagen 1987, 174–86.

62 Leder, *Bugenhagen*, 24.

63 Sehling, *Kirchenordnungen*, VI, part 1, 452–3. Luther held the Florentine hospitals in Italy in high esteem, see his Table Talks, *Luther's Works*, 54, 296.

64 *ibid.*, V, 533.

65 C. Quétel, *History of Syphilis*, Oxford 1990, 50–72.

66 Sehling, *Kirchenordnungen*, V, 360.

67 Rørdam, *Danske Kirkelove*, I, 105–6

68 See 'Huore krancke, mijslige, saare, arme og fattige menneskir schule tracteris oc besørges, een kort vnderwijsning aff Broder Paulus Helie', in *Danske Skrifter af Paulus Helie*, ed. M. Kristensen, III, Copenhagen 1933, 13.

69 *Palladius' Skrifter*, V, 127.
70 See Sehling, *Kirchenordnungen*, VI, part 1, 454; V, 533; Rørdam, *Danske Kirkelove*, I, 105; *Skrifter af Paulus Helie*, III, 26.
71 Rørdam, *Danske Kirkelove*, I, 104; *Skrifter af Paulus Helie*, III, 18.
72 D. Underdown, *Fire from Heaven: life in an English town in the seventeenth century*, London 1993, 90–129. Zwingli's Reformation of Zurich shows a similar pattern, see L. Palmer Wandel, *Always Among Us: Images of the poor in Zwingli's Zurich*, Cambridge 1990.

Chapter 3

Dutch influence on urban planning, health care and poor relief

The North Sea and Baltic regions of Europe, 1567–1720

Jonathan I. Israel

It is arguable that by far the most important external influence on urban planning and improvements – and, as part of this, on health care and poor relief policies – in northern Germany, Scandinavia and the Baltic, from the late sixteenth- down to the early eighteenth century, was that emanating from the Dutch cities. Throughout the northern zone the Dutch factor in the shaping of health care and poor relief vastly exceeded, indeed dwarfed, the impulses emanating from Britain, France or Catholic Southern Europe for more than a century. The object of this chapter is to explain why this should have been so and to attempt to set up a general framework setting out the timing and phases of this crucial impact and the forms which it took.

The first point to grasp is that this widespread adoption of the Dutch example has very little to do with the Baltic bulk trade and the invasion from the early fifteenth century onwards of the Baltic by large numbers of Dutch ships and seamen. As I have argued elsewhere, the general significance – cultural and political, as well as economic – of the Dutch Baltic grain trade has often been exaggerated.[1] It may be true that the Dutch dominated bulk freightage – the commerce in low-value goods, particularly grain, timber and fish – throughout the Baltic and North Sea regions by the middle of the fifteenth century. But this had remarkably little effect on cultural patterns, intellectual life, architectural styles and the like. As far as the traffic in fine goods and high-value materials was concerned, and this is what the merchant elites of northern Germany, Antwerp and London were then chiefly concerned with, it continued to be Lübeck and the Wendish cities which controlled exchange and distribution,[2] and, consequently, it was the civic culture of the Hanseatic cities which dominated the urban cultural context, throughout the Baltic and Scandinavia, as indeed it had throughout the later Middle Ages. As far as urban culture is concerned, Scandinavia remained the backyard of the Hansa cities down to the third quarter of the sixteenth century.

Dutch cultural penetration of the north effectively began only with the migration of thousands of Protestant refugees from the Low Countries in 1567 and subsequent years, with the arrival of the Duke of Alva and the army sent by the king of Spain to crush rebellion and heresy in the Habsburg Netherlands. If the bulk of the refugees who fled east, and north, from the Netherlands settled nearby in the towns of north-west Germany, above all Emden, Wesel and Cologne, smaller but still substantial numbers found refuge further north and east, not only in Bremen, Stade, Hamburg, Lübeck and Danzig, but also in Scandinavia, especially Denmark. By 1575, for example, no less than 14 per cent of the population of Elsinor, the trading town overlooking the Sound, consisted of Netherlands refugees, and their relative level of affluence can be seen from the fact that they were then paying one-third of the taxes collected in the town.[3]

Many of these immigrants, some temporary but others permanent, brought with them not only cash and goods but also varied and often highly specialised skills, so that from around 1570, Dutch influence in the arts and crafts of northern Germany and Scandinavia assumed the proportions of a major cultural factor. But this was just the starting point. It was above all the explosively rapid Dutch conquest of the 'rich trades', the high-value commerce of the North Sea and Baltic regions during the 1590s and opening years of the new century, which ended Hanseatic cultural dominance of the urban cultural context of Scandinavia and the Baltic, replacing it with the cultural hegemony of the Dutch. One by one all the 'rich trades' of the north (except for the time being, exports of English cloth) were taken over by the Dutch, the last to go being Lübeck's control of Sweden's copper exports which was lost to Amsterdam in 1614.[4]

Besides the migration of refugees from the Netherlands, often with valuable skills, and the Dutch conquest of the 'rich trades', there was also a third notable factor which helped shape what I shall term the first phase of Dutch cultural dominance of the urban context of the north, the period from the 1580s until around 1620, namely the responses and adjustments which the Dutch were forced to make in their homeland during the struggle to resist the power of

Spain and consolidate what was, from 1572 onwards, an essentially Protestant revolt. These social and cultural changes wrought by the Revolt were various but the one which, perhaps more than any, had a special relevance to the urban context of the Baltic and North Sea was the building, during the 1580s and 90s, of an entire ring of new fortress towns to shield the fledgling Dutch Republic, extending all the way round from the Ems estuary to Sluis, in States Flanders.[5] Because most Dutch military transportation and supply, like their inland trade, was by water, this phenomenon produced a new kind of integrated urban complex in which fortress, town, harbour and access canals were planned together, classic examples being the towns of Willemstad and Geertruidenberg in northern Brabant and Delfzijl on the Ems estuary. During the first two-thirds of the sixteenth century it had been the Italians who were the leading military engineers and designers of fortifications of Europe. But during the 1580s and 90s, as the struggle in the Low Countries entered a more static phase, it was the Dutch who emerged not just as leading designers of fortifications in Europe but as *the* experts in how to combine fortifications with towns, harbours and waterways. When the Elector of the Palatinate wrote to Prince Maurits of Nassau in 1599, requesting a skilled Dutch military engineer to help design a major new fortress which he was planning, asserting that greater expertise in fortifications was now to be found in the Netherlands than anywhere else in Europe,[6] he was thinking about fortifications alone. But in Hanseatic Germany, Scandinavia and the Baltic, the entire range of Dutch expertise in urban planning was seen to offer exciting new possibilities.

This interest in the whole spectrum of Dutch urban planning was partly due to geography and the great importance in these northern regions of seaborne trade. But it flowed also from the fact that in precisely the period of the arrival of the Netherlands refugees, and the Dutch conquest of the 'rich trades', there was a general quickening and expansion of economic activity, especially in the urban context, throughout Scandinavia and the Baltic. In large part, this was also due to circumstances in the Low Countries. For the closing years of the sixteenth century witnessed a dramatic escalation in Dutch demand for the raw materials produced in these regions of Europe, for military and naval purposes as well as to supply Dutch shipbuilding, commerce and industry. Scandinavian timber, masts, pitch, copper and iron were being shipped to the United Provinces in rapidly growing quantities, and before long

Dutch merchants were also investing in Denmark-Norway and Sweden-Finland, in the production of these materials.

It is therefore not at all surprising that many of the leading Dutch engineers and town planners interrupted their work in the United Provinces from time to time to accept commissions to work elsewhere in the North Sea region and in the Baltic.[7] Simon Stevin, the famous Flemish emigré mathematician and engineer who published a treatise on fortifications, De sterctenbouwing, in 1594, visited Danzig at the invitation of the burgomasters in 1591 and compiled plans for improving and deepening the harbour there, while a few years later he was invited to redesign the harbour and fortifications of Calais. Another leading Dutch engineer of the period, Johan van Rijswijck, having completed the States General's fortifications at Lingen in 1605, travelled to Bremen and Lübeck to take up commissions to redesign the fortifications and harbours of those cities. A third notable figure, Nicolaes van Kemp, was invited to Sweden in 1607 and stayed for three years, planning the harbour and fortifications of Göteborg, a new town founded by the Swedish crown which during the early seventeenth century was virtually a Dutch colony in Sweden.[8]

Nor was it any different in the case of the great Elbe port of Hamburg. In 1609 the Hamburg city fathers, having resolved on an ambitious programme of enlargement and strengthening of the city's fortifications and harbour, invited Johan van Valckenborgh and a group of Dutch engineers to draw up plans and direct the work.[9] This reconstruction of Hamburg's walls, gates and harbour, largely completed between 1616 and 1626 was indeed the most important and extensive remodelling of the city's perimeters of early modern times.

But it was in the Danish monarchy that the importing of Dutch urban planning concepts in this period took place most extensively and fully. It was in the Denmark of Christian IV (1588–1648), an even more avid planner of cities than his Swedish counterparts, that the first phase of Dutch cultural influence in the urban context of the north reached its apogee. A veritable army of Dutch engineers, craftsmen and architects was employed by this, the most ambitious and grandiose of Danish monarchs, in his quest to enhance and fundamentally reconstruct the urban profile of the Danish-Norwegian monarchy. In the years 1606–24, Christian and his Dutch experts rebuilt the entire defensive complex girdling Copenhagen.[10] The first of Christian's new towns, Kristianopel, was founded in 1599 in Blekinge province, today in south-east Sweden, one of the most exposed parts of his monarchy. The town, with its straightened street system was planned along Dutch lines as an integrated whole. His next new town, Kristianstad, was founded in eastern Scania in 1614. This foundation showed almost all the features of the Dutch fortified new towns, with canals being used both to drain and protect the town, and provide access, with the streets geometrically arranged around a central axis linking the two main city gates, and the planning of fortifications and town as an integrated entity.[11] Similarly Dutch in conception and execution was Glückstadt, the new town which Christian founded in 1616 on the Elbe, fifty kilometres downriver from Hamburg, to serve as the main Danish military, naval and commercial base in Holstein. Glückstadt, where a large proportion of the population in the early years was Dutch, was likewise a geometrically calculated, highly integrated combination of fortress, town and harbour in which canals – to drain, protect and provide access to the nearby river – formed a key element.[12] An even more extensive use of canals, this time combined with a fully rectangular grid system, pervaded the plans for Christian's next new town, Christianshavn, founded in 1617 and built during the next decade opposite Copenhagen to the south.[13]

Given this wider context, and borrowing so much from the Dutch, it is only to be expected that the city governments of northern Germany and Scandinavia should also have taken note of, and often borrowed, central features of the new Dutch civic welfare framework. During most of the sixteenth century, whilst bulk freightage remained the main engine of the Dutch economy, urban growth in the Dutch provinces had been undramatic. Amsterdam had grown steadily, but in 1570 was still a city of fairly modest proportions with a population of no more than 30,000. Meanwhile the other Holland cities had hardly grown at all since the beginning of the century; indeed, Leiden, Haarlem, Dordrecht and Gouda were all quite stagnant.[14] Moreover, precisely because bulk freightage provided no basis for large-scale urbanisation, the cities of Holland had felt relatively little of the pressure which faster-growing cities in the southern Netherlands, France, Italy, and central and southern Germany had felt to reform their poor relief and welfare institutions along radically new lines. Indeed, in cities such as Haarlem and Leiden, and to an only slightly lesser degree Amsterdam, very little, down to the closing years of the century, had changed.[15]

Consequently until the 1590s, welfare and poor relief institutions in the cities of the United Provinces were positively backward compared with much of western and central Europe and were decidedly not a model for anyone.

But the very fact that there had been so little reform before the 1590s, combined with the unprecedented explosive growth of the Dutch cities once the breakthrough into the 'rich trades' came, forced the Dutch to undertake much more comprehensive and wide-ranging reforms in poor relief and welfare than could be found anywhere else in Europe at the end of the sixteenth century and opening years of the seventeenth. If, as is clearly the case, it had been a general tendency in Europe since the early sixteenth century to centralise welfare endowments and institutions under civic control, register and support the eligible poor, and discourage begging and vagrancy, once they started in earnest, in the closing years of the century, the Dutch city governments pursued these goals with a determination and resourcefulness such as were to be found nowhere else. If the cities of most of Europe were anxious to curb begging and vagrancy, on the whole they did not succeed. By contrast, in the Dutch context, the measures taken were sufficiently energetic and far-ranging as to be largely (though not totally) effective. The relative absence of beggars and vagrants from Dutch streets, and the link between this and civic welfare policy, was to be frequently remarked on by foreign visitors down to the end of the seventeenth century and beyond.[16] As John Ray expressed it in 1673, 'no Beggars [are] to be seen in all Holland, care being taken to set on work all that are able, and provision made for the aged and impotent'.[17]

In particular, two of the Dutch institutions which took shape at the end of the sixteenth century and beginning of the seventeenth, the *tuchthuis* and the well endowed civic hospital for the disabled and sick poor, seem to have been widely influential in Northern Europe. The *tuchthuis* was an institution serving an entire city, not a ward or parish, much larger and more elaborate than the English workhouse, where facilities were installed which made it possible to concentrate various kinds of specialised and economically valuable (if unpleasant) forms of labour. The Amsterdam *tuchthuis* for men, established in 1595 in a former cloister, became known as the *Rasphuis* because one of the main activities installed there was the rasping of Brazil wood to produce a red dye for the textile industry. The Haarlem *tuchthuis*, established in 1609, was specifically intended as a place where beggars and idle youths removed from the streets could be collected and set to work.[18] There too the rasping of tropical woods, linked to the textile dyeing industry, was one of the principal forms of labour. This concept was then adopted by a number of north German cities in subsequent years, including Hamburg which resolved on, and built, a civic *Zuchthaus* in the years 1615–20.[19] Several features of this institution would seem to confirm that it was closely modelled on the Dutch *tuchthuis,* and not least its size, elaborate organisation, and its name. An English visitor, John Farrington, described it in 1710 as a large establishment 'design'd for the reformation of either sex', where minor delinquents 'are kept to hard labour according to the nature of their crime and former employments, some weaving, some spinning, some rasping logwood' and others, he tells us, beating hemp with a 'wheel... turn'd by men's running in it'.[20] As in Dutch welfare houses and houses of correction, the interior was 'neat and in good order' and adorned with paintings 'suitable to the people there confin'd, as of the Prodigall Son, the Prodigall Son's Return, etc.'. During these same years both Copenhagen and Elsinor likewise each acquired its *tugthus*.[21]

While all medieval towns had had hospices, or a *gasthuis* as it was often called in the Netherlands, where travellers and pilgrims as well as the itinerant poor could lodge, it did not automatically follow that with the Reformation and welfare reforms of the sixteenth century these should be transformed into civic hospitals, directly financed by the city, for disabled and sick poor, where accommodation, medical treatment and medicines were provided free. Indeed, in Hamburg, after the Reformation, it appeared that there was no further use for the *Gasthaus* and it fell into decay and eventually disuse.[22] In Holland, the towns converted their former main hospices into civic hospitals for the poor, a change which required a large financial investment in the 1590s and at the beginning of the new century, but very much as part of their wider welfare policy. In 1592, on taking over financial responsibility for the St Elizabeth's *gasthuis* in Haarlem and providing a permanent income, the city fathers took care to ensure that civic funds were to be spent on maintaining and treating only those sick and disabled whom the city government deemed eligible for admittance. Similarly, at Gouda, it was at the beginning of the seventeenth century that the large, originally fourteenth-century Sint Cathrijne *gasthuis*, still today one of the principal sights of the city (the city museum) was converted into a civic hospital for the poor with a separate section for the mentally ill.[23] These new Dutch civic hospitals were widely noted and probably were a key factor in the revived interest in their former hospices shown by at least some cities in the north during the early seventeenth century. At Hamburg, the city senate decided to rebuild and refurbish the city *Gasthaus* in 1629 but now on a quite different footing from in the past.[24]

Nevertheless, the indications are that borrowing from Dutch civic welfare and health care concepts and institutions in this period, our first phase, was neither so wide-ranging, nor so fundamental in character as was to be the case later. Indeed, I shall argue that, for a number of reasons, the full impact of Dutch civic health care and welfare only manifested itself in northern Germany, Scandinavia and the Baltic after 1648.

One reason for the considerable time lag between the onset of a general cultural primacy in the urban context of Northern Europe (except Britain) at the end of the sixteenth century, and the full impact of Dutch civic health care and welfare policies, was the comparatively modest standing of Dutch medicine itself in Europe down to the 1630s. For although the Dutch universities had begun to flourish and attract foreign students in substantial numbers from the 1590s, the medical faculties were initially far less impressive than much of the rest of Dutch learning and science. But while Dutch medicine only became truly innovative and began to win high regard abroad as late as the 1630s, it made up for this later by retaining its high international standing for several decades after the rest of Dutch scholarship had sunk into decline. The Dutch medical faculties and Dutch clinical practice were undoubtedly the most important, and the most highly regarded, anywhere in Europe during the second half of the seventeenth century, and this golden age of Dutch medicine then continued throughout the first third of the eighteenth century, almost down to the death of the famous Leiden professor Herman Boerhaave (1668–1738).

During the early seventeenth century, consequently, the medical faculties and learned opinion in Scandinavia and Hanseatic Germany by no means took their cues from the Dutch. Swedish medical students, down to the 1630s, studied in Germany, (especially Helmstädt), at Padua, or else at Basel.[25] In the case of the medical faculty at Copenhagen, Basel exerted a remarkable ascendancy which continued for many decades. For over sixty years, from 1577 to

1639, all new professors of medicine at Copenhagen had received their major training at Basel and had Basel MDs.[26] By the 1630s there were numerous Danish students at Dutch universities, at Franeker, Groningen and Utrecht as well as Leiden; but few seem to have studied medicine. Meanwhile, there is no trace of any Swedes studying medicine at Leiden before 1633.[27]

The second reason for the late impact of many Dutch health care and welfare innovations was the general slow-down and suspension of urban projects and development during the Thirty Years' War. This terrible struggle devastated large parts of Germany and severely damaged the economies of many cities. Even those such as Bremen and Hamburg, which escaped unscathed and continued to expand, nevertheless shared in the prevailing sense of insecurity and pessimism, and tended to postpone even quite urgently needed urban extensions, refurbishments and new buildings. Similarly, even though none of the major Dutch cities were sacked or besieged during the second part of the Thirty Years' War (1621–48), they nevertheless felt the pressure and strain of the war, sharing the general uncertainty and postponing major projects until the fighting was over, as Amsterdam did in the case of her new city hall.[28]

Even Denmark-Norway under that frenetic builder Christian IV reflects this suspension of activity, despite the main Danish intervention in the struggle in Germany being of relatively brief duration. The most imposing of Christian's palaces, Frederiksborg, begun in 1599 and built in an obviously Dutch style, was largely complete by 1620, as was the smaller but no less attractive (and obviously Dutch inspired) palace of Rosenborg, begun after the victory of Kalmar, in 1613, on the then outskirts of Copenhagen.[29] The famous exchange, the Børsen, which Christian built in Copenhagen as a headquarters for the city's commercial activity, again adopting a Dutch style, was completed by 1623. After 1623 there were few comparable initiatives except for the reconstruction of Kronborg castle which burned down in September 1629 and had to be rebuilt since it was the fortress which commanded the vital Sound.

After the Peace of Münster (April 1648), the Dutch cities embarked on a new round of urban planning and ambitious development projects. Amsterdam, Leiden, Haarlem, Rotterdam and The Hague not only all put up a remarkable number of new public buildings between the 1640s and 1672, but laid out whole new urban areas complete with canals, streets, bastions and planned housing zones.[30] Leiden replaced all eight of her city gatehouses at this time with larger and more imposing structures. But while the main emphasis was on town halls, churches, gatehouses, civic weigh-houses, admiralty buildings and new canals and housing, a good deal of effort and money was invested also in the enlargement and refurbishing of the welfare establishments, or 'God's houses'. In the 1650s both of the two main orphanages in Amsterdam were rebuilt on a larger scale and with better facilities, which induced most of the minority churches to follow suit, the Walloon congregation commencing their handsome new orphanage in 1669.

At the same time, the cities of northern Germany and Scandinavia embarked on their own programmes of urban development and embellishment and, as part of this post-1648 phase of urban expansion, it was natural that they should borrow many of the remarkable innovations which at that time were being introduced into urban life in Holland. Hamburg, Copenhagen and Stockholm all grew vigorously over the next few decades, and on the one hand laid out new urban zones complete with new harbours, canals and squares; and on the other, saw a need to enlarge and refurbish their welfare institutions. The Hamburg senate rebuilt the *Zuchthaus* after it burned down in 1666, built a *Spinhaus* (1666) or house of correction, for prostitutes and female vagrants, along the lines of the Amsterdam *Spinhuis*, and in the years 1679–81 rebuilt in a considerably larger format the civic orphanage which had been established at the beginning of the century.[31]

Of course, some of the Dutch urban improvements of this period, such as the extension of the system of horse-drawn passenger barges, providing regular passenger services according to published schedules between the Holland towns, a passenger transportation network which reached its zenith in the 1660s, were too specific to Dutch circumstances to be feasibly imitated elsewhere.[32] But others could be, and were, fairly readily adopted. Two of the most notable were the new system of public street lighting which made Amsterdam the first city in history to be lit up in its entirety at night,[33] in 1670, and the new fire-fighting pumps and hoses introduced by Amsterdam in the early 1670s.[34] Adopting the same method as Amsterdam, and importing their lamps from Holland, Berlin and Cologne both lit up their streets with public lamp-posts in 1682.[35] Similarly, the Hamburg fire regulations, published in forty-one clauses in 1685, would seem to show that the whole concept and its technology, based on pumps and leather hoses distributed around the city and stored in designated depots, was modelled on Amsterdam's fire-fighting service.[36] Consequently, there is nothing at all surprising about the fact that, throughout northern Germany, Scandinavia and the Baltic, close attention was paid during these decades to the Dutch innovations in health care and poor relief and that these were the models which were generally followed.

I would argue that there are two main aspects to the increasingly sophisticated civic health care system which took shape in Holland during the second half of the Golden Age. The first has to do with the new medical doctrines and clinical methods being taught in the Dutch universities and at Amsterdam. A number of Dutch professors of medicine and anatomy in this period gained great fame throughout Europe as teachers of applied medicine and clinical method,[37] especially Franciscus de Le Boë Sylvius (1614–72) at Leiden, Frederik Ruysch (1638–1731) at Amsterdam, and again at Leiden, the great Boerhaave. Broadly, Dutch medical doctrine in this period was characterised by a marked stress on applying the principles of chemistry and physics to medicine, great zeal for cleanliness and hygiene, a much more detailed and reliable knowledge of anatomy than had been available in the past, helped by the use of microscopes and new methods of preserving human and animal organs for study, and a strongly empirical approach coupled with a marked lack of respect for traditional medical doctrine.[38] In effect, it was the medicine of the early Enlightenment. In 1699 a senior English physician, Walter Harris, expressed some puzzlement at what he regarded as the peculiar practice of the Dutch to

> bleed so sparingly and seldom as they do. For when they do think fit to bleed, they will seldom or never take away more blood from a man or woman, than we do from an infant of a year old. How they came to fall into such an Extremity of Bleeding little, I cannot well comprehend, considering how profusely the French, and the more southern nations, do use venesection upon most occasions. Nor are the Dutch the most abstemious from Wine and Brandy, which will be apt to heat and inflame the blood, and consequently upon excess sometimes cause diseases that properly require large bleedings; neither am I ignorant that their physicians are very learned men, and must read those excellent books of Galen concerning venesection.[39]

The second factor, possibly even more important than the changes in Dutch medical teaching and clinical practice, was the new administrative and organisational mechanisms created by the city governments, especially Amsterdam, to improve health care and public hygiene. As with the introduction of street lighting and the new fire-fighting system in the 1670s, the strength of city government and its direct participation in administering welfare were crucially important in the reorganisation and improvement of health care. One of the most significant of the Dutch innovations in this sphere, the *Collegium Medicum* at Amsterdam, was set up by the city council in April 1636.[40] Partly the brainchild of Dr Nicolaes Tulp (1593–1674), made famous for us by Rembrandt's painting of 1632 showing him conducting an anatomy class, this institution was originally mainly intended to regulate the apothecaries of Amsterdam. Tulp, who had been a member of the Amsterdam city government since 1622, seems to have had a talent for administration as well as surgery and dissection. Between 1618 and 1636, the number of apothecaries' shops in the city had grown more than threefold, from twenty-one to sixty-six, and the feeling was that more safeguards were needed to protect the public.[41] The *Collegium* consisted of three physicians and two apothecaries and their principal task was to visit all the pharmacies in the city 'two or three times per year', without prior notice, to check that they were not selling impure or bogus medicines and to determine the prices being charged for legitimate supplies. Coupled with this system of *Inspectores*, the city council published a list of authorised prices for medicines, drugs and herbs to which apothecaries were expected to adhere. Henceforth, apothecaries and their assistants were only permitted to practice in Amsterdam if they satisfied the *Inspectores* as to their expertise and probity, and a register of licensed apothecaries was kept.

This system of regulating apothecaries found favour in cities both inside and outside the United Provinces, though there was a time lag of some years before the concept caught on outside the Republic. The city of Bremen published a new civic health *Ordnung*, which was clearly based on the Amsterdam example, at the comparatively early date of 1644, the two chief ingredients of which were the establishing of a system of inspections of apothecaries' shops and the publication of a list of authorised prices for medicines and drugs.[42] Most cities which adopted the system, however, did so rather later. Rostock adopted it, publishing a list of authorised prices for medicines, in 1659.[43] In Stockholm, a *Collegium Medicum* modelled on that of Amsterdam was set up in 1663.[44]

In the early years, the Amsterdam *Collegium* continued to concern itself mainly with the city's apothecaries and the quality and prices of medicines. It was at the prompting of the *Collegium* that the city council decided in 1638 to establish a *hortus pharmaceuticus* in the city where the *Inspectores* could give lessons to apothecaries' assistants in identifying and distinguishing between plants to be used and avoided in the preparing of medicines.[45] In subsequent decades, however, the activity of the *Collegium* was broadened until it was, in effect, regulating most health care in the city, especially with respect to safety, quality and prices. Notable additions to the original concept include the Amsterdam by-law of May 1668, laying down that 'no-one shall be allowed to practice as a midwife in the city unless she has first been examined by the *Inspectores* of the *Collegium* ... and obtained a certificate of expertise' and that of 1675, stipulating as a necessary qualification for securing such a license from the *Collegium*, to have worked as an assistant to a qualified midwife for a minimum of four years.[46] Determined to reduce the rate of infant mortality at birth, the city government was able to use the mechanism of the *Collegium* to ban a number of traditional features of the midwife's craft of which senior medical figures in the city, such as Ruysch, disapproved. The civic regulations on midwifery published in 1682 imposed stiff fines on those who disobeyed the city's stipulations in this respect. These developments too were emulated in the north. After the reorganisation of the Stockholm *Collegium* in 1688, courses in midwifery were instituted there modelled on the courses given by Ruysch in Amsterdam.[47] Johan von Horn, *stadsphysicus* of Stockholm from the early 1690s to 1708 and a key figure both in reorganising the Stockholm *Collegium* and reforming Swedish midwifery along Dutch lines, had trained and worked for no less than twelve years abroad (1679–91), mostly in Amsterdam and Leiden.

An essential part of the culture of civic health care and poor relief in the Dutch context was the close link between city government and the consistories on the one hand, and the management of the 'God's houses'. By concentrating welfare provision together in large central institutions, or in smaller cities, in a single civic hospital, civic orphanage, and so forth, the city councils created institutions with a very large profile in the life of the town and with considerable budgets. This in turn gave them real importance in civic politics and administration. They became emblems of civic pride and were continually visited by outsiders and foreign tourists. In this way achievement of high standards and scrupulous cleanliness on the part of the 'regents' and 'regentesses' who met usually weekly in these establishments to administer them, was seen as a sign of fitness for high position in civic life generally as well as in church affairs. No doubt the Calvinist context and consistory system contributed in some measure to this result. In many cities it was usual for the hospitals to have not just administrators who were close to those running the city, but also one or more sitting members of the city government itself.[48] Thus at Middelburg, the madhouse, installed after the Revolt in a confiscated cloister, was run by four 'regents', the 'president' being one of the city's serving magistrates. The civic hospital at Middelburg was managed also by four 'regents', one of whom, again, was a member of the city council. Nor is this surprising given the funds assigned to the hospital. The city paid the salaries of two university-trained physicians and also several assistant medical staff who were employed to work there full-time. In the case both of the hospitals and the orphanages (which had well equipped sick-wards), concentrating services in large civic establishments made it possible to install a much higher quality of medical care, and better pharmacies, than would have been conceivable had health care been based on small and essentially local institutions. The Dutch system, then, was only practicable in an urban context made up of medium-sized, or large-to-medium-sized cities. It can have had less to offer in the context of a very large city such as London, surrounded by an extensive area virtually devoid of urban areas.

In northern Germany and the few substantial cities of the Scandinavian realms, both the organisational side of the Dutch system and Dutch medical doctrine (including clinical practice) continued to exert a strong appeal until deep into the eighteenth century. From the 1650s onwards until the third or fourth decade of the following century, the medical schools of Sweden-Finland, those of the new universities of Lund, Åbo and Dorpat (closed in 1656 but reopened in 1690 as the *Academia Gustavo-Carolina*) as well as Uppsala, were dominated by professors who had received their principal training in Leiden or another Dutch academy.[49] Of the first fifty physicians appointed as members of the Stockholm *Collegium Medicum* down to 1750, no less than four-fifths – forty –

had acquired at least part of their medical education in the United Provinces.[50] Nor was the sway of Dutch medicine and health care techniques any less overwhelming in the Danish-Norwegian monarchy. It is true that with the steady improvement and expansion of university education in Protestant Germany, Denmark and Sweden-Finland, there was a steep decline in the numbers of German and Scandinavian students studying at the Dutch academies, beginning in the 1670s. Only a small fraction of the number of Danish and Norwegian students studying at the Dutch universities in the 1650s and 60s were still to be found in Holland by the 1690s.[51] But, of all the disciplines for which Dutch academe had become famous, it is quite clear that it was medical studies which resisted the trend most tenaciously, and longest, followed by theoretical science. Voltaire was not far off the mark when he reported to Berlin from Holland in 1737 that between them Boerhaave and the physicist Willem Jacob van 's Gravesande had drawn most, some four or five hundred of the foreign – mostly German – students still to be found at Leiden.[52]

With the rapid decay of the Dutch overseas trading system, industry and economy as a whole from the 1720s onwards, the Dutch cities entered a period of rapid decline and demographic contraction, or at best, as at Amsterdam and Rotterdam, stagnation. Conditions in the Dutch cities visibly began to deteriorate. Without exception, the Dutch academies fully reflected this progressive decay. Still capable of attracting appreciable numbers of German, and a few Scandinavian students in the 1730s, there was a disastrous falling off in the flow of foreign students to Holland in the 1740s.[53] By the middle of the eighteenth century, the Dutch had plainly ceased to be the leading medical nation in Europe; indeed their medical schools were beginning to look less well equipped and furnished with leading medical experts than their counterparts in Germany. At the same time, the cities of the United Provinces, now stripped of most of their former commerce and industry, were no longer a model for anyone. A long and crucially formative era in the history of medicine, health care and welfare generally, in northern Germany, Scandinavia and the Baltic, had come to an end.

ACKNOWLEDGEMENTS

I would like to thank Ole Peter Grell and Robert Jütte for their help with several points discussed in this essay.

NOTES

1 J. I. Israel, *Dutch Primacy in World Trade 1585–1740*, Oxford 1989, 17–36.

2 *ibid.*, 20–1, 27–9.

3 I take these figures from the graph showing immigration from the Netherlands exhibited in the Elsinor town museum. See also A. Tønnesen, 'Helsingørs Udenlandske Borgere og indbyggere ca. 1550–1600', *Byhistoriske Skrifter*, 3, Ringe 1985.

4 Israel, *Dutch Primacy*, 48–52, 96; P.W. Klein, *De Trippen in de 17e eeuw*, Assen, 1965, 328–9.

5 J. I. Israel, *The Dutch Republic: its rise, greatness, and fall, 1477–1806*, Oxford 1995, 262–7.

6 F. Westra, *Nederlandse Ingenieurs en de Fortificatiewerken in het Eerste Tijdperk van de Tachtigjarige Oorlog, 1573–1604*, Alphen aan den Rijn 1992, 66, 76.

7 *ibid.*, 70–6.

8 Israel, *Dutch Republic*, 274; D. Kirby, *Northern Europe in the Early Modern Period: the Baltic world 1492–1772*, Harlow 1990, 239.

9 H. Neddermeyer, *Topographie der Freien und Hanse Stadt Hamburg*, Hamburg 1832, 54–5, 62–5; Carl Schellenberg, *Das Alte Hamburg*, Hamburg 1975, 19.

10 H. Langberg, *Danmarks Bygningskultur. En historisk oversigt*, 2 vols, Copenhagen 1955, vol. 1, 144–5.

11 S. Heiberg (ed.) *Christian IV and Europe. The 19th Art Exhibition of the Council of Europe. Denmark 1988*, Copenhagen 1988, 485, 499.

12 *ibid.*

13 Langberg, *Danmarks Bygningskultur*, vol. 1, 145.

14 Israel, *Dutch Republic*, 114.

15 J. Spaans, *Haarlem na de Reformatie. Stedelijke cultuur en kerkelijk leven 1577–1620*, The Hague 1989, 163–72.

16 C. D. van Strien, *British Travellers in Holland during the Stuart Period*, Leiden 1993, 197.

17 John Ray, *Observations Topographical, Moral and Physiological; Made in a journey through Part of the Low-Countries, Germany, Italy, and France*, London 1673, 52.

18 Spaans, *Haarlem*, 186–7.

19 J. L. von Hess, *Topographisch, politisch-historische Beschreibung der Stadt Hamburg*, 2 vols, Hamburg 1796, vol. 1, 358; Schellenberg, *Das alte Hamburg*, 24.

20 John Farrington, *An account of a Journey thro Holland, Frizeland, Westphalia, etc.,*, 1710, British Library MS Add. 15,570, fo. 88.

21 L. Pedersen, *Helsingør i Sundtoldstiden 1426–1857*, 2 vols, Copenhagen 1936–9, vol. 2, 128.

22 Von Hess, *Topographisch, politisch-historische Beschreibung*, vol. 1, 371–2.

23 J. Schouten, *Gouda vroeger en nu*, Bussum 1969, 100.

24 Von Hess, *op. cit.*, vol. 1, 372.

25 E. Wrangel, *De Betrekkingen tusschen Zweden en de Nederlanden op het gebied van letteren en wetenschap*, Leiden 1901, 298.

26 O. P Grell, 'Caspar Bartholin and the education of the pious physician', in O. P. Grell and A. Cunningham (eds) *Medicine and the Reformation*, London 1993, 78–100, see 88–9.

27 Wrangel, *Betrekkingen,*, 187.

28 Israel, *Dutch Republic*, 863–73.

29 Langberg, *Danmarks Bygningskultur*, vol. 1, 152, 172; V. Wanscher, *Rosenborgs Historie 1606–34*, Copenhagen 1930, 104–12.

30 E. Taverne, *In't land van belofte*, Maarssen 1978, 216, 252–4, 377.

31 Von Hess, *op. cit.*, vol. 1, 358, 363; Schellenberg, *Das alte Hamburg*, 24.

32 This phenomenon has been brilliantly analysed by Jan de Vries in his fine study *Barges and Capitalism*, Wageningen 1978.

33 See L. S. Multhauf, 'The Light of Lamp-Lanterns: street lighting in seventeenth-century Amsterdam, *Technology and Culture*, 26 (1985), 236–52.

34 L. de Vries, *Jan van der Heyden*, Amsterdam 1984, 74–83.

35 Multhauf, *op. cit.*, 250; Leipzig installed 750 Dutch street lamps in 1701.

36 *Der Stadt Hamburg Anno 1685 Neu Revidirte Feuer-Ordnung*, Hamburg 1685.

37 G. A. Lindeboom, *Geschiedenis van de Medische Wetenschap in Nederland*, Bussum 1972, 45, 54–72, 81–4; G. A. Lindeboom, 'Dog and Frog-Physiological Experiments', in Th. H. Lunsingh Scheurleer and G. H. M. Posthumus Meyjes (eds) *Leiden University in the Seventeenth Century: an exchange of learning*, Leiden 1975, 281–91.

38 Initially, this empirical approach was inspired by Cartesian ideas which were deeply entrenched at Leiden by the 1650s but by Boerhaave's time had become purely empirical in character; G. A. Lindeboom, *Herman Boerhaave: the man and his work*, London 1968, 95–101, 366–7.

39 Walter Harris, *A Description of the King's Royal Palace and Gardens at Loo. Together with a Short Account of Holland*, London 1699, 68.

40 Lindeboom, *Geschiedenis*, 79; G. A. Lindeboom, 'Johannes Antonides van der Linden (1609–64), medisch hoogleraar te Franeker en te Leiden', in G. Th. Jensma *et al.*, *Universiteit te Franeker 1585–1811*, Leeuwarden 1985, 358–9. See also W. T. M. Frijhoff, *La Sociéte Néerlandaise et ses Gradués, 1575–1814*, Amsterdam 1981; W. T. M. Frijhoff, 'Non satis dignitatis. . . . Over de maatschappelijke statis van geneeskundigen tijdens de Republiek', *Tijdschrift voor Geschiedenis*, 96 (1983) 397–406.

41 W. H. van Seters, 'De voorgeschiedenis der Stichting van de Eerste Amsterdamse Hortus Botanicus', *Amstelodamum*, 46 (1954), 42.

42 *Eines Ehrenvesten hochweisen Rahts Dero Stadt Bremen Apotheken Ordnung Zu Sampt beygefügter Specification der Medicamenten und deren gerichten Taxa*, Bremen 1644, 4, 15, 29; see also the simultaneously published *Catalogvs Omnium Medicamentorum, tam simplicium quam compositorum et vulgari modo ac chymice praeparatorum, quae in Pharmacopolio Bremensi prostunt cum eorundem taxa seu aestimatione vel precii assignatione*, Bremen 1644.

43 *Verzeichnis Aller so wol Einfachen als Vermischeten auch nach der Chymischen Kunst zugerichteten Artzneyen welche in der Apotheken zu Rostock vorhanden mit beygesetzten billichem Tax und Werth darnach ein iegliches hinfuhro verkauffet werden soll*, Rostock 1659.
44 Wrangel, *Betrekkingen*, 307–8.
45 Van Seters, 'Voorgeschiedenis', 42–3.
46 Caspar Commelin, *Beschryvinge der Stadt Amsterdam*, Amsterdam 1693, 650.
47 Wrangel, *Betrekkingen*, 308.
48 Israel, *Dutch Republic*, 357–8.
49 Wrangel, *Betrekkingen*, 305–6; F. S. de Vrieze, 'Academic Relations between Sweden and Holland', in *Leiden University in the Seventeenth Century*, 345.
50 Wrangel, *Betrekkingen*, 308.
51 S. Veibel, 'Naturvidenskaberne', in K. Fabricius, L. L. Hammerich and V. Lorenzen (eds) *Holland Danmark. Forbindelserne mellem de to Lande gennem Tiderne*, 2 vols, Copenhagen 1945, ii, 289, 317.
52 J. Vercruysse, *Volatire et la Hollande*, Geneva 1966, 36–7, 127.
53 H. T. Colenbrander, 'De herkomst der Leidsche studenten', *Pallas Leidensis*, Leiden 1925, 278–87; H. Wansink, *Politieke wetenschappen aan de Leidse Universiteit*, Utrecht, 1981, 7.

Chapter 4

Continuity and change
Attitudes towards poor relief and health care in early modern Antwerp

Hugo Soly

Few cities in North-Western Europe underwent such dramatic changes in the early modern period as Antwerp, as regards both economic and religious matters. Between 1495 and 1565 Antwerp developed not only into the economic capital of the Low Countries, but it also became the centre of the growing commerce with the rest of the world and took up a leading position in the system of European public finances.[1] The metropolis paid a heavy price for its part in the Revolt of the Netherlands, which resulted in the Spanish Reconquest of Flanders and Brabant. The fall of the city to Parma in 1585, the subsequent blockade of the Scheldt by the Dutch, the emigration of nearly half its population and the flight of capital to the north put an end to Antwerp's 'Golden Age'. During the first half of the seventeenth century the former metropolis continued to play an important role as a centre of production and consumption, but its predominance in international trade was a thing of the past, as the city fathers made clear to the Cardinal-Infante Don Ferdinando in 1635: on one of the stage sets painted by Rubens, Mercury could be seen flying away to make way for *Industria*, which was represented in the guise of the 'Daughter of Poverty'.[2] The commercial decline was indeed only partly compensated for by the expansion of the luxury industries. From the 1650s onwards, local producers had in addition to cope with growing competition, both from within the Spanish Netherlands and outside it, which threatened to lose the city its last trump card.[3]

The year 1585 was also a turning point from the point of view of religion. In spite of the Heresy Laws of Charles V and Philip II, the Antwerp city authorities had always adopted a pragmatic and tolerant attitude towards the Jews and the followers of the 'new religion', with the exception of the Anabaptists who distanced themselves from the establishment and who were mainly drawn from the lower social orders. The relative tolerance of the city fathers was owed in large part to economic motives: severe repression would have damaged the commercial interests of the metropolis, since many businessmen were to be found among the 'heretics'.[4] During the third quarter of the sixteenth century Antwerp developed into one of the bulwarks of international Protestantism, culminating in the revolutionary years of 1577–85, when the Calvinists held the political and military reins. The impact of the Reformation can be deduced from the lists of the Citizens' Guard which were drawn up immediately after the capitulation of the city: the 11,000 or so adult men were almost equally divided between Protestants and Catholics.[5] The 'heretics' were given four years in which to convert or to leave. The overwhelming majority fled the city, for both religious and economic reasons. Anyone who stayed and did not come over to Catholicism exposed themselves to all manner of persecution, risked paying heavy fines and became uneligible for poor relief. It is therefore not surprising to learn that the zeal for conversions among the Catholic clergy bore fruit. By 1648 Antwerp had transformed itself into a bulwark of the Counter-Reformation, a place where Anabaptists or Lutherans were no more to be found and where Calvinists remained in such small numbers that the authorities considered them completely harmless.[6]

It is clear that the meteoric rise of Antwerp as a cosmopolitan international port, and the subsequent transformation of the metropolis into a more closed, orthodox society with a much narrower economic base had repercussions on the patterns of social and cultural relations. Both before and after 1585, the city fathers and the ecclesiastical authorities were conscious of the fact that large numbers of the city's population lived in abject poverty. However, it does not follow from this that the upper and middle classes perceived the social problem in the same way, nor that their motives for setting up welfare facilities and instigating health care measures were identical.

The current situation in research does not permit all the relevant questions to be answered. Little is known about long-term changes in the employment structure and the distribution of wealth. There is a lack of studies on marriage patterns and family types, on the demographic and social consequences of epidemics, on medical practice, on relatives and neighbours as sources of help, on the wider solidarity networks, on crime and many other aspects of life in the city that might shed light on developments in poor relief and health care provision. Nevertheless, despite this dearth of information, we can draw a few outlines.

SOCIAL POLICY IN A COSMOPOLITAN WORLD-PORT

The extraordinary economic expansion in Antwerp between 1495 and 1565 acted not only as a magnet for merchants and skilled craftsmen coming from all over Europe, but also attracted thousands of impoverished country-dwellers hoping to find work in the metropolis. In consequence of this influx, the population *intra muros* increased from some 40,000 to more than 104,000. The available evidence suggests that Antwerp was able to assimilate large numbers of immigrants, who constituted the overwhelming majority of its population, and that demographic expansion did not create serious tension between natives and newcomers. Yet the urban economy did not continuously keep pace with the increasing population. During the periods 1526–35 and 1551–8 many merchants and industrial entrepreneurs had to cope with economic difficulties resulting from wars and structural changes in the transit trade, during all of which the demand for workers declined while the supply of labour continued to rise, which brought about under-employment and even unemployment.[7]

The sources that enable us to throw some light on the distribution of wealth present us with some stark contrasts. Four out of every five inhabitants were not able to contribute anything to the enforced loan of 1574. An analysis of the monthly property tax raised from November 1584 to April 1585 also reveals gross inequalities: the propertied classes represented only 24 per cent of the total population; the others were too poor to be able to pay anything.[8] In other words, economic growth and social polarisation went hand in hand. The triumph of commercial capitalism offered many businessmen hitherto unknown opportunities for making themselves rich, and also made it possible for other residents such as high officials, members of the professions and artists to prosper as well – but it led to the proletarianisation of numerous master craftsmen and the impoverishment of wage labourers.

The problem for craftsmen with few financial resources in sixteenth-century Antwerp was not so much trying to reach the status of master as maintaining their economic independence. In the most labour-intensive branches of the textile industry this was even more difficult, since on the one hand the rising demand for exports tempted both merchants and the better off master craftsmen to try and get round the corporate restrictions on the size of an enterprise by subcontracting work, and on the other hand the growing membership and recurring crises undermined the negotiating position of small producers. This is the reason why only fifty of the eight hundred master silk weavers belonged to the propertied classes.[9] The expansion of sub-contracting in the construction industry produced similar effects: in the mid-1580s, four out of every five master masons and master carpenters were too poor to pay any taxes.[10]

It is not possible to investigate whether there were any significant differences in employment between the various occupational groups, between the Antwerp-born and the immigrants, and between men and women. However, even on the assumption that three of the four or five family members were employed for the whole year, there is no doubt that the average proletarian family often had difficulty in making ends meet. Of course, there were employees who ran little risk of descending into poverty because they earned exceptionally high wages, like the printers and compositors, but such groups were in the minority. For the bulk of the working population the 'Golden Age' was in fact an 'Iron Age'. It is true that almost all categories of wage labourers in the metropolis towards the middle of the century earned more than their colleagues in other towns and cities of the Low Countries, but that does not detract from the fact that their standard of living had also deteriorated. Between 1500–10 and 1550–60 the wages of construction workers in Antwerp rose by about 75 per cent, whilst the price of grain, the staple food, increased by more than 150 per cent. Moreover, nowhere was living space so expensive as in the metropolis: by 1560 domestic rents had more than trebled, which meant that an unskilled worker would have to pay out at least 15 per cent of his annual income for an extremely humble dwelling. Add to this that the excise duty on beer, the principal drink of common folk, had also risen substantially and it becomes understandable why large numbers of wage labourers increasingly had to tighten their belts.[11]

Taking all this into account, it is not surprising that the charitable institutions that had come into being in the late Middle Ages found themselves completely unable to cope by the second quarter of the sixteenth century. Although we lack precise details, there can be no doubt that the number of people in need increased considerably in the metropolis. This can be seen from the complaints of the almoners – rich citizens entrusted by the city administration with responsibility for the distribution of public assistance funds – about the growing imbalance between requests for relief and the available funds on the one hand, and on the other, the attempts of the aldermen radically to reduce the numbers of beggars on the streets.[12]

The much harder attitude towards beggars, both in Antwerp and in other towns and cities of the Low Countries, was concurrent with changes in the perception of poverty. Since the late Middle Ages the urban upper classes had made a distinction between the deserving and the undeserving poor, i.e. between people whose destitution could be ascribed to 'natural' or 'accidental' origins like widowhood, illness, disability, old age or having a large number of children to feed, and those who could not cite such reasons to explain their impoverished circumstances; able-bodied beggars in particular were presented as anti-social individuals who had scant regard for the moral values of their fellow citizens and who chose of their own free will to live on the fringes of society.[13] During the first half of the sixteenth century however, greater use was made of such stereotypes, and not merely to discriminate among the poor and to stigmatise social categories. Through the image of the 'sturdy beggar', who was characterised as the incarnation of idleness, disobedience and godlessness, the city authorities also justified the enactment of laws that criminalised all forms of beggary and the introduction of new systems of civil relief. The explanation for this must be sought in a combination of two factors.

On the one hand the gradual deterioration in living conditions in many rural areas was inducing more and more men and women to leave the villages of their birth, which meant that migratory movements were assuming greater significance, which increased fears of disturbances to public order. From the 1520s onwards the city magistrates were increasingly confronted with growing social and political unrest. Initially the agitation was limited to food riots, among the destitute, but before long it included skilled labourers, who began to organise strikes, and even to master craftsmen, who protested against the imposition of new *aides*.[14] The situation was becoming all the more dangerous because the collective actions were coupled with anti-clerical movements, as can be seen from the spread of Lutheranism and Anabaptism.[15]

On the other hand, numerous urban employers noted that beggary was on the increase, while they themselves had difficulty in finding cheap labour. This was an apparent paradox, inherent in the uneven development of capitalism, but both the merchant-entrepreneurs and the well established master craftsmen only saw that the 'meeting' of capital and labour was going anything but smoothly. This was the reason they translated the growing social problem into moral terms. They were convinced that able-bodied beggars had only themselves to blame for their misery and that the generosity of the charitable institutions only encouraged idleness.

It is in this context that the reorganisation of urban poor-relief has to be situated. On 31 January 1525 the magistracy of Mons drew up a plan, which in December of the same year was taken over word for word by their counterpart in Ypres and immediately put into practice. The new system was based on three principles: a strict interdiction on begging, the obligation for all able-bodied persons to work regardless of age or sex, and a centralisation of the existing relief funds into a 'common box' to make it possible to select and control those in need. Thenceforth only the following categories were considered eligible for civil relief: the poor who were not able to work – thus the aged, the sick and the disabled; families who had fallen into poverty through misfortune and who were ashamed of their current situation; and finally, all those who needed temporary help either because they had a large number of children or because of 'accidental' circumstances.[16]

The transition from medieval charity to a social policy in the real sense of the word meant that the local authorities took on responsibility for all 'respectable' citizens who ended up in need. It does not follow from this that the latter had a right to civil relief: they could only hope that their social superiors would practice Christian good neighbourliness. The idea that poor relief was essentially a task for the civil authorities in any case gave a new dimension to relations between the public and private domain.

In 1526 Juan Luis Vives gave a thorough, ideological justification for the actions of the urban magistrates. The civil authorities had to be responsible for poor relief, as he maintained in his *De Subventione Pauperum*, because they had a duty to maintain public order. If the poor were abandoned to their fate, then those who were well off ran great risks which could bring down the whole urban community. The city fathers had to make good citizens of the beggars by imposing on them an obligation to work or to support them if they were unfit to do so. By forbidding begging they stimulated the urban economy moreover, since the possibilities for employment would increase, and at the same time they would put the poor in a position to subject themselves to God's will and to fulfill their social obligations.[17]

Prominent Catholic theologians like Christiaan Kellenaer and Jacob de Pape, who had initially supported the opposition of the mendicant orders to the new social policy, quickly revised their opinion. The few clerical voices that were still being raised to protest against municipal legislation to control begging were put to silence in January 1531, when the theological faculty of the Sorbonne decided that the reorganisation of poor relief at Ypres was in accord with the scriptures, the teachings of the Apostles and the laws of the church.[18] Eight months later the Emperor Charles V promulgated an ordinance in which he encouraged municipal welfare reforms in the Low Countries.

However, the rise of centralised poor relief systems cannot be ascribed to such interventions. It was the trend towards social disruption as a consequence of economic and demographic changes and everything related to them in the political and religious domains that drove more and more municipalities to follow the examples of Mons and Ypres: Lille in 1527, Nieuwpoort and Oudenaarde in 1529, Valenciennes and (probably) Bruges in 1530, Bapaume, Hesdin and Saint-Omer after 1531, Ghent in 1535, Breda in 1536, Brussels in 1539, Antwerp in 1540, Louvain in 1541 and Malines in 1545.[19] It was not purely by chance that all these towns belonged to the county of Flanders or to the duchy of Brabant, the most densely populated and most urbanised provinces in the Netherlands, nor that most of them were centres of industry. The new social policy offered not only the opportunity to discipline the destitute and to punish the indolent: it could also be used as an instrument to enforce low-paid work.

It was precisely for this reason that the reorganisation of poor relief in Antwerp leant support to the aspirations of both the upper and the middle classes. In 1532 the aldermen stipulated, referring to the imperial decree, that thenceforth no-one, with the exception of the mendicant friars and the lepers, could beg for alms again, and that any destitute persons who had lived in the city for less than one-and-a-half years had to leave the city.[20] They did, however, delay creating a common box, because almost all the charitable institutions – including the Tables of the Holy Ghost, the parish poor relief organisations – were in the hands of private individuals or were controlled by the clergy. The only exception was the *Kamer van de Huisarmen*, founded in 1458, whose control rested in the hands of officially appointed almoners. When in 1540 the latter declared that, owing to a lack of funds, they were no longer in a position to fulfill their task, the city fathers finally decided that the income of all the charitable institutions was to be handed over to the *Kamer*, with the exception of the Saint Elisabeth Hospital, the leper house at Terzieken and the homes for the elderly founded by various craft guilds.[21]

It is easy to understand why the almoners pressed for a reorganisation of poor relief and why they were met with a positive response: they belonged to the upper echelons of the business community and they were expected to make up any deficit incurred by the *Kamer*, which meant an ever greater drain on resources since the funds being distributed increasingly exceeded income. Although Pope Julius II approved the initiative of the Antwerp magistracy, the administrators of the Tables were less than cooperative, so that the welfare reform threatened to fail. It was only after the Governor-General of the Netherlands had put them under pressure that they agreed to the creation of a common box and handed over their funds to the *Kamer*.[22]

Laicisation did not mean that the interests of the clergy were ignored – quite the opposite. The aldermen and the almoners were aware of the fact that social control and ecclesiastical discipline overlapped. This is why they stipulated that pub-crawling would automatically lead to removal from the poor lists and that public sinners would not be eligible for civic relief; this applied particularly to adulterers. The recipients of outdoor relief had to produce a 'confession token' for the almoners at least once a year, and prove that they had fulfilled their Easter duties.[23]

It seemed that the new social policy was producing the desired effects. The magistracy adhered strictly to the interdiction on begging: during the third quarter of the sixteenth century, no less than 2,335 idlers were arrested, i.e. five times as many as in the period 1525–49.[24] For their part, the almoners used rigorous criteria to determine who would be eligible for outdoor relief. This can be deduced from the testimony they produced in the middle of the 1560s: growing poverty obliged them to provide support for ever increasing numbers of families, whose numbers had risen to a thousand.[25] If we assume that the families involved each had three or four members, then the permanent dole-drawers represented 3.5 per cent to 4.5 per cent of the civilian population *intra muros*, excluding foreign traders and their households. This low figure is corroborated by the following calculation: between 1560 and 1569 the annual income of the *Kamer* from collections and gifts came to an average of 6,800 Brabant pounds,[26] which made it possible to provide some 3,450 persons each with the daily equivalent of one kilogram of rye bread, i.e. about 10 per cent of the earnings of an unskilled male labourer.

Although the almoners continued to repeat that they could only support a small portion of the needy because of a lack of funds, the *Brede Raad* (literally 'Broad Council') – which included both rich burghers and guild officials – refused to provide subsidies. We cannot divine their motives, but everything seems to indicate that two considerations played a role here. On the one hand, they defined the social problem in moral terms, as has already been remarked, which substantially meant that poor relief in their opinion ought to be reserved for those whom they considered to be respectable members of the local community, who conformed to the standards and values of their social superiors and whose destitution could not be ascribed to personal failings. This explains why the very old and the very young were over-represented among the recipients of outdoor relief,[27] and why citizens who made gifts or legacies for the benefit of the poor usually stipulated that the money should go for the care of foundlings, orphans, the aged or the sick. On the other hand, the interdiction on begging and the exclusion of the able-bodied poor made it possible to keep wages down, or at least to prevent their increase in accordance with inflation. From the employers' point of view the timing of the poor relief reform was perfect, since the 1540s were characterised by accelerated economic growth and, in consequence, a growing demand for labour.

To argue that the value system of the middle and upper classes played a decisive role in the selection of the destitute for relief is not to deny that the foundlings, the orphans, the aged and the sick constituted a social problem in themselves. The combination of population growth and impoverishment raised the likelihood of the spread of infection and led to family disruption, with the consequence that more and more individuals fell through the meshes of the informal social networks and became dependent on institutional care. Those who were admitted to an orphanage or hospital could count themselves lucky, at least from a material or medical standpoint. All the more so, because they formed a small minority. Although Antwerp in 1555 counted no less than 1,500 foundlings and abandoned children, the new asylum – built in 1523 – could only accommodate fifty girls and boys. All the others were fostered, usually with peasant families close to the metropolis; they came to the institution, which had its own physician, only if they were ill.[28] Gifts and legacies from rich burghers made it possible for the almoners to found two orphanages, one in 1552 for girls over the age of eleven (the *Maagdenhuis*) and one in 1558 for boys over the age of twelve (the *Knechtjeshuis*). After extensions during the 1560s, each of the two new orphanages was able to accommodate about a hundred children. Each had its own schoolteacher and surgeon. The girls had to sew or make lace until they reached the age of twenty. The boys were given training in tailoring, shoemaking, pin-making or cooperage. After their eighteenth birthday they had to leave the institution and go into service with a master craftsman; some of them were given a study bursary and sent to the University of Louvain, but they were the exception.[29]

What was the situation for the elderly lacking sufficient means or a charitable family? Around 1500, Antwerp had sixteen small hospitals where the elderly could enjoy free board and lodging. Six of them, however, had been founded by guild officials of the furriers, curriers, shippers, mercers, cloth-dressers and smiths, so that they were only available to members of those organisations, in particular for masters or their widows. The capacity of the other hospitals was very limited: together they could house only sixty women and some thirty men. The preponderance of widows became even greater in the sixteenth century, since the eight new hospitals set up between 1504 and 1562 together provided accommodation for fifty women and twenty men at most. The figures show that the capacity of these did not keep pace with the demographic expansion and the growing extent of poverty. The available information suggests moreover that most of the inmates came from the lower middle classes rather than the ranks of the wage earners.[30]

If they fell ill the poor could summon the doctors and surgeons who worked for the city council; medicines were paid for by the almoners.[31] If their physical condition required institutional care, then the patients were sent to St Elisabeth's Hospital. The statutes of this institution stipulated that all sick residents of Antwerp who were destitute would be eligible for admission, with the exception of the lepers and those who were suffering from chronic or incurable diseases. The nuns who ran the hospital also refused many other patients, usually through lack of space, though often too for moral reasons which applied in particular to people who had had venereal disease or to pregnant women; admitting the latter, according to the religious, would be considered by unmarried women from the lower classes as an encouragement to sinful living.

Despite building a second ward in 1507–10 (which made it possible to separate male and female patients) and a number of smaller extensions in later years, the capacity of St Elisabeth's was totally insufficient. Towards 1560, the institution housed about a hundred beds, i.e. one per thousand inhabitants. This low ratio – in contrast with the situation in Bruges, where it was 3:1000 – explains why two and sometimes even three patients had to share the same bed, as can be seen from the number of inmates, which during the 1550s and 60s always came to more than two hundred per day. If we assume that the average stay in the hospital was the same as in the eighteenth century – namely 52 days – then about 1,400 paupers must have been admitted every year.

It is doubtful whether the patients were better off in the hospital than in their own lodgings. The reports that the Bishop of Cambrai and the almoners drew up in the middle of the century show that the inmates were not particularly pampered. The nuns left everything to maidservants, who went about their work in such a slovenly manner that 'patients who had been in the hospital once would rather die than return there', as the magistrate declared. The inmates not only had to do without medical attention, but they had to be content with a scant diet consisting mainly of peas, beans and other 'rough' foodstuffs, and in addition they had to contend with dreadful conditions of hygiene. The situation only improved after the Bishop appointed a new Mother Superior in 1551, raised the number of religious to twenty-four and dismissed all the maidservants. However, the patients received even less meat and fish than before the reform and remained dependent for their medical treatment on the doctors and surgeons working for the municipality, since the hospital still had no physicians of its own.[32]

Apart from St Elisabeth's Hospital, there were few institutions of any medical consequence in sixteenth-century Antwerp. Lepers had to remain outside the city walls, where they found shelter in the cloister of Terzieken, and after 1552 in eighteen small houses which had been erected at the city's expense in the hamlet of Dambrugge. Although the metropolis was afflicted by epidemics on several occasions – which according to contemporaries claimed many victims, especially in 1512, 1529, 1557 and 1571 (probably 1700 deaths) – the magistracy never took energetic steps to stop the spread of contagious diseases. Since the plague houses dating from the late Middle Ages were far too small, the almoners had to send the poor who had suffered from the pestilence to St Elisabeth's, where they often lay next to the other patients, since the hospital's *Pestilentiehuys* could only accommodate a few patients.[33] Impoverishment and family disruption may have led to the expulsion of a growing number of real or alleged pauper lunatics. In 1553 the almoners found it necessary to build a madhouse, where such patients could be locked up. There was no mention of any medical treatment; anyone who was not amenable to reason or who caused serious disturbance was simply put in chains.[34]

It is clear that the poor had not lived through any 'Golden Age'. The new system of outdoor relief introduced in 1540 left most of them out in the cold, since the destitution of growing numbers of wage labourers was not defined as a social problem. Even individuals and families whose plight continued to arouse sympathy increasingly ran the risk of slipping through the formal safety net, since the growth of institutional care lagged far behind demographic expansion. Of course, the creation of a common box did not prevent religious orders from continuing to distribute alms, just as the interdiction on begging did not put an end to uncontrolled forms of private charity. However, the large-scale arrests of beggars and vagabonds show that personal alms-giving and begging was considered unacceptable and potentially dangerous by the city authorities. It seems reasonable to suggest that, as far as the labouring poor are concerned, informal social networks based on the principle of reciprocal exchange ought to be accorded great importance. Unfortunately, the available evidence is not conclusive enough to permit us to say anything about the degree to which paupers in sixteenth-century Antwerp could rely on relatives, neighbours and other local networks for mutual support.

WELFARE PROGRAMMES IN A CALVINIST REPUBLIC

During the Revolt of the Netherlands, which broke out around 1568, there was a steady influx of artisans and wage labourers, among whom were many Calvinists, from Hainaut, Artois and Flanders. But there was also a reverse flow of people who left the metropolis for economic or religious reasons, so that its population declined to 82,000 in 1585. Although the political upheavals, military operations, naval blockades and steep tax rises undermined the position of Antwerp as a port for world trade, the level of employment remained high because of changes in the urban economy which shifted labour from trade to manufacturing and from old to new industries. The revolutionary years 1577–85, when the Calvinists held power, were witnesses of a spectacular growth in the production of silk fabrics and fine linens. Towards 1585 the textile industry provided a living for more than 13,000 men, women and children – i.e. 16 per cent of the total population.[35]

The administrators of the Calvinist Republic had good reasons for wanting to maintain the existing poor relief system. First and foremost, earlier developments such as the prohibition of begging, the collection of alms by civic officers, and the centralisation and reallocation of funds were in line with the attitudes towards the poor taken by Protestant reformers. Second, the new authorities had to take into account the fact that half the population consisted of Catholics and that they were most strongly represented amongst the low-income groups. Consequently, the Calvinists had every interest in showing themselves to be reasonably tolerant on religious matters and in leaving in peace those clergy who performed socially useful functions.

It should also be noted that the numbers of poor as a whole fell between 1577 and 1584, in both absolute and relative terms, because industrial growth led to full employment and even to wage rises while grain prices remained low, which meant that most proletarian families enjoyed an exceptionally high standard of living.[36]

This happy situation and the non-discriminating attitude of the Calvinist almoners, who distributed alms without asking the religious convictions of the recipients, explains why the annual income of the *Kamer* from collections and gifts was on average

50 per cent more than in the 1560s,[37] although the number of inhabitants in the meantime had dropped by almost 20 per cent.

The fact that the Calvinist almoners continued the social policy of their Catholic predecessors does not mean that everything remained as before. Laicisation and rationalisation were now much higher on the agenda. All religious orders were forbidden to distribute alms and their support funds were handed over to the common chest. The nuns of St Elisabeth's Hospital had to put themselves under the supervision of the civil authorities, who released them from their monastic vows and obliged them to wear a 'secular habit'. Much more attention was paid to the poor's sick and invalids. The almoners appointed two surgeons with exclusive responsibility for the medical treatment of the needy, and they engaged numerous women to deal with those who had scabies or other skin diseases on a regular basis. They also planned for the creation of a second hospital and a number of plague houses, but the political and military events hindered the realisation of these projects.[38]

While it is true that the obligation to work had been the basic principle of social policy in Antwerp ever since 1540, the Calvinists attempted to combine social and moral discipline with economic gains in a more systematic way. The boys' orphanage was transformed into a manufactory and the best qualified inmates thenceforth had to work for merchant-entrepreneurs; the redundant boys were apprenticed to master craftsmen.[39] Some textile manufacturers even received permission to pick up young idlers, both boys and girls, 'out of the gutter' and put them to work in their establishments.[40]

PATTERNS OF CHARITY IN A CATHOLIC INDUSTRIAL TOWN

After 1585 there were two developments that gave a new dimension to public and private charity. In the first place it was no longer international trade that functioned as the engine of the Antwerp economy, but the manufacture of luxury goods – which meant that quality and artistic creativity occupied places of far greater importance than previously. For this reason, skilled craftsmen and artisans who had sufficient capital and credit acquired hitherto unknown opportunities for social advancement – at least until the middle of the seventeenth century, since after that time many trades endured a long period of stagnation or even deteriorated drastically.[41] In the second place, the establishment of a new spiritual order went hand-in-hand with changes in the perception of poverty, which now came to be associated much more strongly with religious values. The Jesuit Franciscus Costerus – whose monumental series entitled *Katholieke Sermoenen*, published between 1598 and 1616, exerted a great deal of influence[42] – once more latched on to the medieval idea of evangelical poverty: the poor were the keepers of the gates of Heaven, where they awaited the coming of those who had practised the Christian love of fellow men and women. The poor had earned their eternal happiness by accepting their lot with patience and by working hard – since work was a religious duty, a way to worship God. The rich for their part could only earn their place in Heaven by carrying out good works, which in concrete terms meant that they had to give alms and that they could not use the presence of sinners in their midst as an excuse for shunning beggars. However, they could not go to the other extreme and so overload the able-bodied needy with charitable gifts that they would be led into the temptation of abandoning their religious and social duties.[43]

In order to understand the basis and extent of the social problem, a distinction should be made between skilled and unskilled workers on the one hand and between the first and the second half of the seventeenth century on the other. After the capitulation of the city, all categories of wage earners had a number of years of terrible hardship; but between 1590 and 1620 their material conditions improved, because the demand for labour increased much more quickly than the number of inhabitants (from 42,000 to 54,000), which led to wage rises while the prices of essential foodstuffs went down.[44] During the following three decades however, the growth of employment lagged behind the growth in the population. The consequences were to be seen mainly in a variety of unskilled and semi-skilled occupations, where over-supplies of labour produced chronic underemployment or unemployment; the situation of the families involved was worsened by an upward trend in the price of domestic rents and grain. Towards 1650 destitution had reached such proportions that 'even the stones would weep if the tears that daily fell upon them could bring them to life', as the almoners wrote to the city authorities.[45] In spite of the application of ever stricter selection criteria, about four thousand inhabitants out of a total of 63,000 (i.e. more than 6 per cent) were eligible for outdoor relief.

Although quantitative information is lacking, there can be no doubt that the extent of poverty during the second half of the seventeenth century became even greater. It is true that the cost of living went down, but this gain did not compensate for the loss of income brought about by the growing unemployment among adult men, whether skilled or unskilled. Some guild-based industries held their own and there were even branches that expanded, but the general picture was one of decline. This can be deduced from the growth of lace manufacture, which reflected a lack of alternative employment opportunities, since laceworkers were very badly paid.[46] Since the charitable institutions were being forced deeper into debt, the clergy considered it advisable to reconsider its attitude towards the problem; with evangelical poverty in the background, emphasis was laid to an increasing degree on the existence of a large number of 'undeserving poor'.

The centralised system of poor relief was maintained, but it was no longer able to contribute to the regulation of the labour market, because most employers needed skilled craftsmen. It does not follow from this that the profitable employment of paupers was lost sight of. In 1613 the magistracy of Antwerp followed the example of Amsterdam, Gouda and other towns and cities in the Dutch Republic by opening a *Dwinghuis* ('House of Correction') with the purpose of locking up the 'sturdy beggars' and setting them to work. The city administration hoped not only to be able to train idlers through enforced labour to become useful members of urban society, but also indirectly to exert pressure on the price of labour by encouraging the poor to work for employers at the lowest possible wage from fear of ending up in an institution governed by a severe regime. To encourage such initiatives, the central government in 1617 promulgated the principle of obligatory labour for all able-bodied poor, to cover the whole country. The city fathers of Brussels and Ghent also erected prison workhouses during the 1620s, but they soon realised, as did their colleagues from Antwerp, that such institutions did not deliver the expected economic advantages. In consequence, support for obligatory work quickly waned. Within a few decades the majority of the inmates no longer consisted of beggars and vagrants, but of 'debauched' persons, children in particular, who at the request of their families were put under lock and key to avoid scandal.[47] The only other attempt made in seventeenth-century Antwerp to combine charity with economic profit was the installation of a large workshop in 1664 in the boys' orphanage, in which silken yarns were wound on to reels. This initiative was taken in support of the needs of the silk-manufacturers, who mobilised large numbers of women and children to carry out such badly paid work.[48]

The exhortations of the Archdukes Albert and Isabella to raise a poor tax when the finances of the charitable institutions were no longer sufficient met with a negative response however. At the end of the seventeenth century the city fathers of Antwerp did raise an 'entertainment tax', of which the yield would be destined for the poor, but they made no attempt to oblige the better off citizens to contribute to civil relief. However, they enthusiastically put the articles from the ordinance of 1617 and the decree of 1618 into practice: these stipulated that the needy had to be supported by the charitable institutions of the place in which they were born or where they had been residing for at least three years.[49] They also followed the advice of the Archduchy to replace the private pawnshops with a public loan office. Such *Bergen van Barmhartigheid* designed by Wenceslas Cobergher on the model of the *Monti di Pietà*, were set up in fifteen towns and cities of the Spanish Netherlands between 1618 and 1633. Unlike their Italian counterparts however, they did not in the first instance give loans to the poor, as can be seen from the high rates of interest (12 to 15 per cent) they charged.[50]

Although poor relief remained the responsibility of the lay authorities, the clergy exerted a far greater influence than hitherto. In 1608 the Archduchy accorded the bishops the right to examine the annual accounts of all the charitable institutions, and in 1609 they endorsed the decision of the synod of Malines, according to which the needy who had not performed their religious duties had to be excluded from civil relief – in the first instance for three months, and if they did not mend their ways it would be forever. Some years later the central government did, it is true, stipulate that the supervision of the charitable institutions and the appointment of their administrators were the prerogatives of the sovereign, but in practice a growing number of foundations escaped the direct control of the civil authorities, which led to numerous conflicts with the clergy, both in Antwerp and in other towns and cities of the Spanish Netherlands.[51]

The triumph of the Counter-Reformation produced a number of positive effects with regard to charity. Although the Antwerp magistracy had given its attention during the sixteenth century to the education of pauper children, the number of schools to which they could go remained very limited. Since the post-Tridentine clergy considered (re-)education to be the spearhead of its religious and moral programme, successive bishops of Antwerp between 1592 and 1611 stimulated the foundation of Sunday schools where children who had received no kind of schooling could learn the principles of the Catholic religion and the rudiments of reading. By 1620 the Sunday schools, which were also subsidised by the city authorities, had some 3,200 pupils aged between seven and fifteen. Their success must be seen in context however, since the distribution of bread for most parents was the chief motive for sending their children to these institutions where the emphasis lay on catechism classes.[52]

The clergy could usually expect a positive response to their exhortations to exercise charity, anyway. The total value of the collections, gifts and legacies for the benefit of the poor rose considerably, both in absolute and relative terms, at least to about 1650, after which the charitable drive gradually lost momentum.[53] Just as in the sixteenth century, the members of the elite remained mainly concerned with the very young and the very old, likewise between 1594 and 1656 the wealthy burghers erected no less than twelve new hospitals for the elderly which together could house sixty-three women and thirty-eight men.[54] The inscription on the memorial plaque which one of their founders, the merchant Cornelis Lantschot, had erected in the Church of Saint-Jacob throws some light on their motives: *Men wint de Hemel met geweld, Of is te koop met kracht van geld* – 'Heaven can be won with the strength of the sword, or bought with the power of gold'.[55]

Important changes took place in the field of health care provision. It is true that the capacity of St Elisabeth's Hospital remained inadequate. The decline in population raised the ratio of beds to inhabitants to a mere 1.5:1000 – still a very low figure, especially if account is taken of the fact that the hospital had to take large numbers of wounded soldiers, in particular from 1621 to 1647 and during the last quarter of the seventeenth century. The patients could, however, look forward to improved care, not only because the number of nuns was brought up to thirty, but also and above all because from 1595 there was a permanent medical staff present at all times. This was thanks to the Portuguese merchant Simon Rodriguez d'Evora, who provided the Mother Superior in 1594 with the necessary finance to appoint a physician and two surgeons on a permanent basis. The first candidates were chosen by d'Evora himself, but thereafter the right to appoint them fell to the magistracy, which paid a portion of their salaries. In principle, the physician and the surgeons could only treat patients who had a legal address in Antwerp and moreover, the same doctors had to pay for their own medicines, plasters and salves. Serious cases could only be examined by the physician, who was also obliged to take responsibility for all major operations.[56]

Through lack of detailed information it would be risky to make any generalisations, but it could be assumed that the medical practice in St Elisabeth's Hospital measured by seventeenth-century standards left little to be desired, since the successive doctors enjoyed an unrivalled reputation. Lazarus Marcquis, who was in charge from 1606 to 1617, not only did medical research, but also published a treatise in Dutch about the plague in order to make it clear to the authorities and the public at large what the symptoms were and what measures could be taken to combat it.[57] In 1620 he was the driving force behind the foundation of the *Collegium Medicum*, which thenceforth supervised the practice of medicine in Antwerp and organised examinations for surgeons, apothecaries and midwives; similar institutions were subsequently set up in Brussels (1649), Ghent (1663) and Courtrai (1683).[58] The successors to Marcquis also gained celebrity not only at local level but also outside Antwerp. This was particularly true of Michiel Boudewijns, who had first studied philosophy and theology and then medicine, which explains why in his publications he paid attention both to religious and moral problems as well as medical practices, including hygiene and diet. In some respects he was a man of the Counter-Reformation, as can be seen from his judgement that a doctor could not be obliged to treat heretics, but in other fields he took a less doctrinal view: a doctor had to condemn prostitution, though under certain conditions he could prescribe prophylactics to counter venereal diseases; *abortus provocatus* was strictly forbidden, but in the case of illness all means were permissible to save the life of a pregnant woman. It was probably under the influence of Boudewijns that the bishop of Antwerp commissioned the Mother Superior of St Elisabeth's to set up a large pharmacy.[59]

The treatises in which Marcquis and other doctors encouraged the authorities to take measures to counter the plague had some effect. In 1604, 1625, 1636 and 1658 several plague houses were built at the cost of the city with the purpose of keeping infected patients under quarantine. The new institutions were not able to take in all the victims, but the magistracy also took stringent precautions: persons and goods from towns where plague had been reported were not allowed to come into the city; the meat and fish markets were systematically supervised; a 'dog killer' was appointed to destroy all freely roaming animals; it was forbidden to buy or sell objects from plague-infested houses. Yet these administrative and policing measures fell far short of what was required and plague continued to devastate the city. Plague manifested itself for the last time in Antwerp in 1668, but ten years later another infectious disease made its appearance, probably a form of pernicious influenza, which caused no less than six thousand deaths – i.e. almost 10 per cent of the total population.[60]

Finally, it should be noted that pauper lunatics in the public madhouse still received no medical attention whatsoever. The only innovation resulted from the enlargement of the madhouse between 1645 and 1648 which led to the construction of a number of individual cells. The continuing rise in the number of inmates – from forty in the 1620s to more than eighty at the end of the century – cannot be ascribed to a changed attitude on the part of the elite towards mental illness, since the *simpelen*, the harmless lunatics, retained their special place in the annual procession.[61] Perhaps the explanation is to be found in the impoverishment of more and more families.

NOTES

1 H. van der Wee, *The Growth of the Antwerp Market and the European Economy, Fourteenth–Sixteenth Centuries*, 3 vols, The Hague 1963.

2 See J. C. Gevartius, *Pompa Introïtus... Ferdinandi*, Antwerp 1642, after 146. See also the comments by J. R. Martin, *The Decorations for the Pompa Introïtus, Ferdinandi*, Brussels 1972, 178–9.

3 For a detailed analysis, see A. K. L. Thijs, 'De nijverheid', *Antwerpen in de XVIIde Eeuw* , Antwerp 1989, 131–51.

4 On this topic, see the important study by G. Marnef, 'Antwerpen in Reformatietijd. Ondergronds protestantisme in een internationale handelsmetropool, 1550–77', 2 vols, PhD thesis, Louvain University 1991, to be published in English by Johns Hopkins University Press; and the article by the same author 'The Changing Face of Calvinism in Antwerp, 1550–85', in A. Pettegree, A. Duke and G. Lewis (eds) *Calvinism in Europe, 1540–1620*, Cambridge 1994, 143–59.

5 Calculations based on F. J. van den Branden, 'De Spaansche muiterij ten jare 1574', *Antwerpsch Archievenblad*, XII (s.d.), 217–88; and R. Boumans, 'De Getalsterkte van Katholieken en Protestanten te

Antwerpen in 1585', *Belgisch Tijdschrift voor Filologie en Geschiedenis*, 30 (1952), 741–98.

6 A. K. L. Thijs, *Van Geuzenstad tot Katholiek Bolwerk. Maatschappelijke betekenis van de Kerk in contrareformatorisch Antwerpen*, Turnhout 1990; M. J. Marinus, 'De Protestanten te Antwerpen, 1585–1700', *Trajecta*, 2 (1993), 327–43.

7 van der Wee, *Growth*, II, 144–66, 209–22; P. Daems, 'Private Huizenbouw te Antwerpen, 1526–50', Ghent University 'Licentiate' thesis, 1976; H. Soly, 'De Schepenregisters als Bron voor de Conjunctuurgeschiedenis van Zuid- en Noordnederlandse Steden in het Ancien Régime', *Tijdschrift voor Geschiedenis*, 87 (1974), 529–38.

8 For more detail, see J. Van Roey, 'De Correlatie Tussen het Sociale-Beroepsmilieu en de Godsdienstkeuze te Antwerpen op het Einde der XVIde Eeuw', in *Bronnen voor de Religieuze Geschiedenis van België. Middeleeuwen en moderne tijden*, Louvain 1968, 239–57.

9 A. K. L. Thijs, *Van 'werkwinkel' tot 'fabriek'. Detextielnijverheid te Antwerpen, einde 15de en begin 19de eeuw*, Brussels 1987, 189–201, 219–36.

10 H. Soly, *Urbanisme en Kapitalisme te Antwerpen in de 16de Eeuw. De stedebouwkundige en industriële ondernemingen van Gilbert van Schoonbeke*, Brussels 1977, 195–282.

11 For greater detail, see the important studies of E. Scholliers, *Loonarbeid en Honger. De levensstandaard in de XVe en XVIe eeuw te Antwerpen*, Antwerp 1960, and 'De lagere Klassen', in *Antwerpen in de XVIde Eeuw*, Antwerp 1975, 161–80.

12 Antwerp, Stadsarchief, *Privilegekamer*, no. 914, f° 31, 63v°-64, 71v°, 92v°, 101, 141v° .

13 See the useful comments by H. Pleij, *Het Gilde van de Blauwe Schuit. Literatuur, volksfeest en burgermoraal in de Late Middeleeuwen*, Amsterdam 1972; and P. Vandenbroeck, *Jheronimus Bosch. Tussen volksleven en stadscultuur*, Berchem 1987.

14 See especially A. Henne, *Histoire du règne de Charles-Quint en Belgique*, 10 vols, Brussels and Leipzig 1858–60, *passim*.

15 van der Wee, *Growth*, II, 143–53.

16 J. Nolf, *La Réforme de la Bienfaisance Publique à Ypres au XVIe siècle*, Ghent 1915; P. Heupgen, 'La commune Aumône de Mons du XIIIe au XVIIIe Siècle', *Bulletin de la Commission Royale d'Histoire*, 90, (1926), 319–72; and his *Documents Relatifs à la Règlementation de l'Assistance Publique a Mons du XVe au XVIIIe siècle*, Brussels 1929.

17 For a detailed analysis, see H. C. M. Michielse, *Secours van den Aermen*; Jan Luis Vives, 'De Hervorming van de Armenzorg rond 1525 en de Opkomst van een Andragogische Technologie', *Tijdschrift voor Agologie*, 15, (1986), 267–87.

18 J. Decavele, *De Dageraad van de Reformatie in Vlaanderen, 1520–65*, 2 vols, Brussels 1975, I, 126–9.

19 See C. Lis and H. Soly, *Poverty and Capitalism in Pre-Industrial Europe*, Brighton 1981, 89.

20 Antwerp, Stadsarchief, *Privilegekamer*, no. 914, f° 164–5.

21 Antwerp, Stadsarchief, *Vierschaar*, no. 1823; and *Kerken en Kloosters*, no. 2105.

22 Antwerp, Stadsarchief, *Kerken en Kloosters*, no. 2111; E. Geudens, *L'Hôpital St Julien et les Asiles de Nuit à Anvers depuis le XIVe Siècle jusqu' à nos Jours*, Antwerp 1887, 35–7, 168–71.

23 Antwerp, Stadsarchief, *Privilegekamer*, no. 914, *passim.*; E. Geudens, *Le Compte Moral de l'An XIII des Hospices Civils d'Anvers*, Antwerp 1898, LXXI–LXXII.

24 X. Rousseaux, 'L'Incrimination du Vagabondage en Brabant (14e–16e siècles). Langages du droit et réalitès de la pratique', in G. Van Dievoet, Ph. Godding and D. van den Auweele (eds) *Langage et Droit à Travers l'Histoire. Réalitès et fictions*, Louvain and Paris 1989, 159–63.

25 Geudens, *Compte moral*, L.

26 Antwerp, Openbaar Centrum voor Maatschappelijk Welzijn, *Kamer van de Huisarmen*, registers. I would like to thank Mrs Kathy Haemers, who is presently preparing a 'Licentiate' thesis on private charity in early modern Antwerp, for providing this information.

27 See, for instance, E. Païs-Minne, 'Weldadigheidsinstellingen en ondersteunden', in *Antwerpen in de XVIde eeuw*, Antwerp 1975, 191–3.

28 Antwerp, Stadsarchief, *Kerken en Kloosters*, no. 2110; E. Geudens, *Recherches Historiques sur l'Origine des Hospices des Aliénés et des Enfants Trouvés à Anvers*, Antwerp 1896, 7–10.

29 E. Geudens, *Van Schoonbeke en het Maagdenhuis van Antwerpen*, Antwerp 1889; and his *Het Antwerpsch Knechtjeshuis*, Antwerp 1895.

30 Païs-Minne, 'Weldadigheidsinstellingen', 188–9 (with references to the literature on this topic).

31 Geudens, *Compte moral*, , LXXI.

32 P. De Commer and H. Soly, 'Harde Tijden voor Zusters en Zieken, 1490–1585', in *Het St-Elisabethziekenhuis te Antwerpen: 750 jaar Gasthuis op 't Elzenveld, 1238*, Brussels 1988, 70–4, 82–3, 87–90.

33 See especially A. F. C. van Schevensteen, *La Lèpre dans le Marquisat d'Anvers aux temps passés*, Brussels 1930; and his *Documents pour Servir a l'Etude des Maladies Pestilentielles dans le Marquisat d'Anvers jusqu' à la Chute de l'Ancien Régime*, 2 vols, Brussels 1931.

34 Païs-Minne, 'Weldadigheidsinstellingen', 187; D. Verhelst, *Geschiedenis van de Psychiatrische Zorg in Antwerpen*, Antwerp 1991, 6.

35 Thijs, *Van 'werkwinkel' tot 'fabriek'*, 159–70.

36 Scholliers, *Loonarbeid*, 141–3.

37 See note 26.

38 Geudens, *Compte moral*, XXXIV; De Commer and Soly, 'Harde tijden', 74–5.

39 Geudens, *Antwerpsch Knechtjeshuis*, 70–3.

40 A. K. L. Thijs, 'Een ondernemer uit de Antwerpse Textielindustrie: Jan Nuyts, ca. 1512–82', *Bijdragen tot de Geschiedenis*, 51, 1968, 63–5.

41 H. van der Wee, 'Industrial Dynamics and the Process of Urbanization and De-Urbanization in the Low Countries from the Late Middle Ages to the Eighteenth Century: a synthesis', in Idem (ed.) *The Rise and Decline of Urban Industries in Italy and the Low Countries (Late Middle*

Ages–Early Modern Times), Louvain 1988, 349–51; Thijs, 'De nijverheid', *passim*.

42 H. Storme, *Preekboeken en Prediking in de Mechelse Kerkprovincie in de 17e en 18e eeuw*, Brussels 1991, 52–61.

43 Thijs, *Geuzenstad*, 203–4.

44 Scholliers, *Loonarbeid*, 143–6; and his 'Peilingen naar de Conjunctuur en de Koopkracht', *Antwerpen in de XVIIde eeuw*, 153–67.

45 Quoted in Geudens, *Compte moral*, LIII.

46 Thijs, *Van 'werkwinkel' tot 'fabriek'*, 238–41, 244, 252.

47 L. Stroobant, 'Le Rasphuys de Gand', *Annales de la Société d'Histoire et d'Archéologie de Gand*, III (1898), 240–71; A. Hallema, 'Het Antwerpsche Tuchthuis, een Hollandsche Navolging', *Antwerpsch Archievenblad*, 2nd series, VI (1931), 3–26; Cl. Bruneel, 'Un épisode de la Lutte contre la Mendicité et le Vagabondage: la maison de correction *(tuchthuys)*, de Bruxelles', *Cahiers Bruxellois*, 11 (1966), 29–72; F. Mahy, 'De Brugse Tuchthuizen in de 17de en 18de Eeuw. Een onderzoek naar hun maatschappelijke functie', 2 vols, Ghent University 'Licentiate' thesis, 1982.

48 Geudens, *Antwerpsch Knechtjeshuis*, 104–5; Thijs, *Van 'werkwinkel' tot 'fabriek'*, 177–83, 355–8.

49 Geudens, *Compte moral*, LIV–LV, C–CI; Bonenfant, *Le problème du Paupérisme en Belgique à la Fin de l'Ancien Régime*, Brussels 1934, 90–1.

50 P. Soetaert, *De Bergen van Barmhartigheid in de Spaanse, de Oostenrijkse en de Franse Nederlanden, 1618–1795*, Brussels 1986, 89–102, 190–1, 207–10.

51 For a general survey of the literature, see G. Maréchal, 'Het Openbaar Initiatief van de Gemeenten in het Vlak van de Openbare Onderstand in het Noorden van het Land Tijdens het Ancien Régime', in *Het Openbaar Initiatief van de Gemeenten in België. Historische grondslagen (Ancien Régime). Handelingen van het 11de Internationaal Colloquium, Spa, 1–4 September 1982*, Brussels 1984, 510–12.

52 K. de Raeymaecker, 'Aspecten van de Contra-Reformatie te Antwerpen in de Zeventiende Eeuw', in *Antwerpen in de XVIIde Eeuw*, 79–80; E. Put, *De Cleijne Schoolen. Het volksonderwijs in het hertogdom Brabant tussen Katholieke Reformatie en Verlichting, eind 16de eeuw – 1795*, Louvain 1990, 25–6, 104–5.

53 See note 26.

54 De Raeymaecker, 'Aspecten', 78; See also Geudens, *Compte moral*, 20–85.

55 Quoted in R. Baetens, *De Nazomer van Antwerpens Welvaart. De diaspora en het handelshuis De Groote tijdens de eerste helft der 17de eeuw*, 2 vols, Brussels 1976, I, 301.

56 A. F. C. Van Schevensteen, *Les Chirurgiens de l'Hôpital Sainte-Elisabeth à Anvers jusqu'à la Fin de l'Ancien Régime*, Brussels 1927, 43–4; Baetens, *Nazomer*, I, 224–6; De Commer, 'Oude en Nieuwe Problemen, 1585–1796', in *Het St- Elisabethziekenhuis*, 122–35.

57 C. Broeckx, 'Notice sur le Docteur Lazare Marcquis', *Annales de la Société de Médecine d'Anvers*, 13 (1852), 5–35; A. Goovaerts, 'Lazare Marcquis', *Biographie Nationale*, 13, Brussels 1894–5, 562–73.

58 M. van Roy, 'De Medische Verzorging in Vlaanderen tijdens de 17e en 18e eeuw', in R. van Hee (ed.) *Heelkunde in Vlaanderen door de eeuwen heen. In de voetsporen van Yperman*, Brussels 1990, 126–33.

59 C. Broeckx, 'Eloge de Michel Boudewyns', *Annales de la Société de Médecine d'Anvers*, 6 (1845), 5–34; J. P. Tricot, 'De Geneeskundige Zorgen', in *Het St- Elisabethziekenhuis*, 138–40.

60 Van Schevensteen, *Documents*, 110–233; F. Janssens and E. van Cauwenberghe, 'Crisis en Bevolking te Antwerpen rond het midden van de 17de Eeuw', *Bijdragen tot de Geschiedenis*, 60 (1977), 262–6, 269.

61 Verhelst, *Geschiedenis*, 7–9, 12.

Chapter 5

Health care provision and poor relief in early modern Hanseatic towns
Hamburg, Bremen and Lübeck

Robert Jütte

CONCEPTS

For centuries it has been recognised that poverty is often accompanied by illness or its social and economic consequences. Despite health insurance and welfare programmes, disease and its effects remain numerically important as a cause of poverty up to the twentieth century. In an age which did not yet know a national health service or any other form of compulsory health insurance, the effects of prolonged illness or sudden death during an epidemic were disastrous. It meant the bringing down of the formerly self-sufficient lower income groups to the ranks of the destitutes. When victims recovered, they emerged ensnared in debts incurred during their malady. Epidemic diseases incapacitated at least as many people as they killed, thus reducing income and assets as well as leaving bereaved children and spouses in their wake.

In this chapter I examine the awareness of the social and economic importance of illness in three Hanseatic cities during the early modern period, including for good reasons also the eighteenth century, which saw the most important changes in health care provision in Germany before the rise of the modern welfare state at the end of the last century. In what follows, I first discuss the care of illness at home, analysing the provision of free medical care and medicines to the sick poor. This type of health care needs to be understood as part of a larger system of support of domestic economies in an environment in which disaster, be it illness or unemployment, might occur at any time. In addition to the medical care for the domiciled poor there were various poor relief institutions which had their own medical staff and which offered both in- and out patient care for the sick poor.

OUTDOOR RELIEF

The direct tie between poverty and disease, or rather between disease and impoverishment did not, however, escape comment by contemporaries. Even the poor law reformers of the sixteenth century, who argued most forcefully for a strict prohibition of begging and a system of discrimination and deterrents in the granting of relief, acknowledged that the sick poor were a special case, as for example Andreas Hyperius (1511–64), a prominent Protestant theologian whose tract on poor relief *De Publica in Pauperes Beneficentia* (Latin version published posthumously in 1570; English translation 1572) was not only carefully studied on the continent but in Elizabethan England as well. He also delivered an expert opinion on poor relief reform which influenced the reorganisation of poor relief in the city of Bremen in the second half of the sixteenth century.[1] In the English translation of his tract Hyperius argues that the citizens

> universally desire, that beggers, especially valiant and able of body, may bee brought in order: and that the true pouertie, that is, such as are diseased by age, sickness or other casualty mai be prouided for: and fynally that some certaine way maye be prescribed for the right expending and disposing of the common almes.[2]

Similar ideas were expressed by Johannes Bugenhagen (1485–1558), another Protestant reformer and theologian who set up or revised the Poor Ordinances in many north German towns.[3] It must be remembered that Bugenhagen's schemes were not limited to poor relief but extended to the entire church reorganisation. The famous *Kirchenordnung* adopted in Hamburg in 1529, is considered the classic expression of his social ideas. The early church orders and poor law ordinances on which Bugenhagen put his stamp have been viewed almost exclusively from the vantage point of what they say about larger themes of the Reformation, in particular the dissolution of the monasteries, the re-evaluation of charity and the opposition to mendicancy. Yet these documents also represent often the only description of the civic programme of health care provision for the needy and the fullest statement of the town council's intention for the poor. They delineate some of the magistrate's goals and help us to map the categories by which the poor were to be evaluated and located within the context of religious and social values of a civic community undergoing important changes.

Let us take the example of Hamburg, where as early as 1522 evangelical teaching had been introduced.[4] By 1527 three of the city's four principal pastors were adherents of Martin Luther. Already two years before Bugenhagen's Evangelical Church Order was promulgated for Hamburg, the parish of St Nikolai had taken the first step toward recasting parochial relief in an evangelical mode by creating a *Gotteskasten*, which was modeled on Luther's 'common chest'.[5] Money from this fund was to be used for the benefit of the parish poor who had become indigent 'through no fault of their own, but rather as the result of God's inscrutable will'.[6] In December 1527 the three other parishes also established their own common chest and elected their own poor relief officers (deacons). These important changes were confirmed and institutionalised by the Hamburg Church Order of 1529 which included a special and detailed section on how to deal with the funds set aside in the common chest for the relief of the poor. The article entitled *Welcker Armen ut der Casten Besorget Scholen Werden* gives, for example, a general list of those who should be given alms. It addresses first the indigent 'resident poor' (*husarme*) and then refers to the diligent artisans and workers who could not make a living. Third-listed were those poor who due to sickness or physical disablement (*de dorch krankheit edder feil erer litmaten nichtes vorwerven konnen*) had become destitute.[7] The article concludes by describing exactly the network of parish officers through which the local and alien poor applying for alms could be screened. Similar criteria for discriminating among the poor can be found in the Church Orders of other north German cities. According to the Church Order of Lübeck (1531), for example, aid should also be given to poor foreigners who fell ill while staying in the city.[8] In such a passage Bugenhagen and his followers were doing little more than echoing Luther's principles of poor relief issued in his famous 'Letter to the Christian Nobility of the German Nation' of August 1520 and the poor relief scheme he devised for the little Saxon town of Leisnig in 1523.[9]

It was not the intention of either Hyperius or Bugenhagen, chief architects of the new poor law in north German towns, that the sick poor be subject to conditions intended to force the idle, the imprudent, or the drunken out of begging into productive labour. Both conceded that sickness, disability and old age rendered some of the labouring poor unable to support themselves and their families.

Such misfortunes were not to be blamed on the destitute themselves, who were held entitled to alms, or even better, to assistance in their own homes, and were to be taken into special institutions (hospitals, almshouses, etc.) only at their own request.

It was the special fear of epidemic and endemic diseases which directed the eyes of the magistrates to that particularly endangered section of the population, the poor. Plague was most fatal in overcrowded suburbs where the lower classes lived. Bills of mortality and eye-witness reports show the epidemics originating in the poorest suburbs. The town physician Johann Böckel, for example, advised the aldermen of the city of Hamburg in 1597 what to do in times of plague. In his opinion the plague was breaking out in some of the poorest quarters and then being spread to other areas of the town by beggars roaming the streets.[10] Not surprisingly, a frequent result of this linkage between plague and the poor was a marked increase in repressive measures directed not only against vagabonds but also against the native indigents. Visiting homes following notification, isolating those who were suspected of being plague carriers and building plague hospitals – all followed, as the local government and its health authorities began to aim at the lower classes.

Although the plague struck with an unusual ferocity, it was – like the other virulent epidemics – in quantitative terms a less important threat to the family economy than the daily burden caused by common diseases. A prolonged illness or a permanent physical debility could, more than anything else, push an individual or a family over the narrow boundary between poverty and indigence. For if someone in good health had problems in making ends meet, the incapacity to work aggravated their already precarious financial situation and social dislocation was likely to ensue. It is therefore important to keep in mind that it was not primarily the cost of health care (help by non-professional healers was sometimes equally expensive!) which quickly used up the small savings or other financial and social resources of the population at the lower end of the economic scale. When the main earner was sick, it became more difficult for a family to raise money for the ordinary cost of living. And when the person died on their sickbed the dependants had to find a livelihood and were often forced to pay off debts incurred during previous episodes of illness. In eighteenth-century Hamburg, for example, a pamphlet describing 'A scheme for the advantages of the sick poor of this place'

(*Plan zum Vortheil der hiesigen kranken Haus-Armen* published in Hamburg in 1779) describes a typical case of a family father falling ill. He first tries to get help from professional healers. When that fails he turns to quackery. His poor state of health goes from bad to worse. Finally he dies and leaves behind his wife and several children. The widow tries desperately to make a living until she too is worn out and follows her husband to the grave. In the meantime some of the children have also died – children who, as the anonymous author of this treatise puts it, 'could have become useful members of the republic'[11] if their father had not died in the first place. However, one has to be careful not to generalise the scanty and sparse information on the disease conditions and physical disabilities of the poor. From the limited observations which we have on eighteenth-century Hamburg and/or other early modern German cities (e.g. Cologne[12]) it should be clear that the study of the interrelationship of disease and poverty must take into account the pre-disease economic status of the individual and the nature of the disease itself. The impact of disease is not the same for everybody, not even for those who belong to the so-called 'lower classes'. But the difference depends also on the nature of the disease, as a future social history of epidemics will surely demonstrate.

Finally, and of greatest interest in the present context, is the fact that the relation of public authority to the sick poor, the most frequent recipient of poor relief, changed during the early modern period. The clearest indicators of the altered relationship between the sick and the state were the various new medical aid schemes for the poor adopted by some Hanseatic towns in the second half of the eighteenth century. Ultimately, the goal of medical relief was the prevention of impoverishment. A 'Report On the Care of the Sickness' from 1781 for the local authorities of the city of Hamburg, pointed out that 'if one let all our paupers recite the stories of their misfortunes, at least half of them would name an illness as the direct cause [of their misery]'.[13] A study on poor relief in eighteenth-century Cologne reveals that 37 per cent of those who requested public relief in 1798 mentioned illness ('krank') as principal cause for their poverty.[14] In Lübeck, the preacher Johann Hertel in 1792 also arrived at the conclusion that there were strong links between disease, illness, accidents and poverty. In particular he refers to diseases caused by bad housing conditions, suggesting that the crowded and humid living quarters (known as *Gänge*) should be torn down.[15]

That Hanseatic towns saw sickness as a vital element in any effective scheme for the relief of the poor is shown by the inclusion of details of the state of health in the questionnaire for the poor relief officers in Hamburg in 1788. Not only in this Hanseatic town but also elsewhere, health care provisions for the poor developed gradually into 'an ambitiously conceived, far-reaching program that sought to weed out one of the tap roots of poverty: unforeseeable, capricious illness'.[16] By the end of the eighteenth century, beginning with infants and children, poor law authorities were offering medical services on a large scale to both the sick and the well in the hope of preventing future disease or disability.

INDOOR RELIEF

There can be no doubt that the provision of some sort of medical care for the poor did already exist in late medieval and early modern Hanseatic towns. The respective schemes depended upon a variety of local factors such as religious forces, political considerations, economic pressures, inherent necessities, the scope of bureaucratic intervention and the vested interests of the medical profession.

Like in other early modern German towns there was a twofold system of health care for the urban poor. One was institutionalised medical care in hospitals, asylums, workhouses and orphanages; the other was the supply of free medical aid in the form of seeking out and paying for the advice and remedies of surgeons, physicians or apothecaries. In the early modern period illnesses attended at home greatly outnumbered poor patients treated and cared for in hospitals or similar institutions. This was understandable, given the scarcity of hospitals and the Christian model of the care of the sick within the family, which was favoured by the well off. For a very long time no fully fledged system existed for aiding the sick poor on a regular basis, other than extra payments for special needs and for medical care during a bout of sickness. Still, it seems safe to argue that free medical care available to the poor already played a major role in the relief of the poor in Hamburg, Bremen and Lübeck before the introduction of special medical relief schemes for the poor in these Hanseatic towns during the eighteenth century.

Already in the first half of the sixteenth century, German town councils instituted a centralised or decentralised system of outdoor relief, which although probably inadequate, gave rise to several historically important changes. From that time onwards we have an increasing number of records which indicate the intensification of local government relief to medically indigent persons. This is the case, for instance, in the city of Bremen, where the common chest established in 1534 was also in charge of the sick poor, providing them with medical attention and medicines.[17] During the later part of the sixteenth century we uncover further proof of how early magistrates had recognised that sickness was a major cause of pauperism and destitution. In Bremen, for example, we notice a determination to extend medical aid also to the non-registered poor.[18] Already the Church Order of 1534 had made no difference in helping foreign and local poor in case of sickness, despite the fact that normally residency was among the principal criteria for eligibility. The first ambitious and far-reaching program of medical aid to the non-registered poor was, however, introduced for the first time by the city of Hamburg. But this was not until the 1790s.[19]

There can be no doubt that even the poorest members of the community availed themselves of expert help, and the various municipal poor relief agencies in Bremen, Hamburg or Lübeck do not seem to have objected to their seeking out the professional care available in the medical marketplace at that time. The money given by the deacons or *Gotteskastenverwalter* to pay for medical aid was not given automatically or as a right. The poor had to petition for it. And it was left to the poor relief officers assisted by medical professionals to judge whether someone was medically indigent and qualified for free medical aid. During the Thirty Years' War, a poor relief officer by the name of Cordt Carstens drew up a special list of all the sick poor in the city of Bremen. Those registered sick poor received special payments every Monday.[20] In Bremen as well as in the other towns included in this study, the deacons and poor relief officials seem to have been flexible in their response to the needs of the poor, and sickness was one of most frequent reasons for temporary increases in weekly allowances and for extra payments to cover expenses for medical treatment. Occasionally a sick poor would be sent to an eye doctor (*Starstecher*), a lithotomist (*Steinschneider*) or a bonesetter for special treatment which was often rather expensive. Account books also often refer to other forms of medical relief – trusses, water cures, treatment for the 'French Pox', crutches and bleeding. In Hamburg and Bremen the overseers of the poor sometimes hired transport to assist the sick poor.[21] Midwifery expenses were often paid, too. It also happened that poor relief recipients were enlisted in caring for other sick poor in cases of old age and terminal illness.

It is often difficult to separate 'medical' relief from the rest. The majority of the poor (broken families, the elderly and unwed mothers) received some kind of medical care or another as an integral part of their welfare support. A close look at the account books of the poor relief agencies in Bremen, Hamburg or Lübeck reveals that neither recipients nor relief officers normally made any clear distinction between health care and poor relief.[22] There were many poor householders who received at the same time or consecutively a combination of food, fuel, lighting, clothing, nursing care and free medical treatment while they were on the dole. The group among the poor which received free medical aid or special sick benefits only was usually quite small. However, when war or epidemics struck a city, the number of sick poor in need of relief could come close to that of the registered poor who received regular allowances for a variety of reasons, listed in the account books simply as 'poor' or 'in distress'. This happened, for example, in Bremen in 1539 when the nearby countryside had been hit by a flood and had left many peasants destitute,[23] or in 1626–7, when there was a large influx of refugees into this Hanseatic town because of the Thirty Years' War. At the same time the already rather strained situation was even further aggravated by the plague.[24]

With a few exceptions, the three Hanseatic towns did not provide medical aid to the poor on a contract basis, as was the case in many English towns. They either employed state-salaried medical[25] and public health officers or paid annual lump sums to practitioners who treated the poor. In some cases towns switched from one system to the other. In seventeenth-century Bremen, for example, the parochial poor relief officers were obviously dissatisfied with the contract system and therefore joined together in order to employ a surgeon on a full-time basis. A certain Master Hinrich was supposed to treat free of charge as many patients as he could handle.[26] The high demand for such medical services was occasionally met by the willingness of individual physicians and surgeons who treated poor patients for the love of God.[27] Where this voluntary medical relief did not exist, the poor law authorities had no other choice than to appeal to the doctors' Christian conscience. This happened, for example, in Bremen during the Thirty Years' War. In 1634 the deacons who were in charge of poor relief turned to the local church authority for help. They suggested that the ministry should ask the medical profession for gratis cooperation. They argued that if every doctor or surgeon in the city would pledge to supply free medical care for one month on a rotation basis, the General Relief could do without the full-time surgeon who cost them a lot of money which could then be used for other pressing needs. Unfortunately we do not know what happened to this interesting plan which counted on the civic responsibilities of medical practitioners.

In 1750 the physician Anton Heins was asked by the magistrates of the city of Hamburg to make suggestions for an improvement of medical policing, as the number of quacks, empirics and unorthodox healers in Hamburg was obviously very high and many irregularities in medical practice had occurred which threatened to undermine the health of the citizens. Heins published his proposal two years later. He argued, for example, that restricting different types of medical practice to those qualified for them would improve the general standard of medical care and would lead to a better provision of health care for all inhabitants. Heins, in fact, recognised that many people could not afford to consult a proper physician and therefore turned to quacks. He recommended that physicians and surgeons hold special office hours for the poor (*Armensprechstunden*).[28]

In 1768 several physicians volunteered to supply free medical care and medicines to the poor for a period of two years. The scheme was to be supported by subscriptions, which would go towards buying medicines for the sick poor. After some months the experiment failed but the initiators did not give up. In 1778 many of the same people founded the *Institut für Kranke Hausarme*, which was later on incorporated into the General Poor Relief as its medical branch.[29] Seven physicians (Deuterich, Gericke, Jänisch, Leppentin, Nootnagell, Ulffers and Weiss) seem to have been involved in proposing the scheme. They were assisted by four surgeons and five apothecaries, one for each parish. The money which was necesssary for making up prescriptions and distributing them without payment was collected by two eminent and well known citizens, Pastor Sturm and Professor Büsch. The first published 'Report' by the Hamburg Medical Relief took pride in its achievements by pointing out that 'so many people have ... been cured'.[30] Within the first two years, 1,170 sick poor had been treated within the framework of this new scheme. There were 926 cured, 152 died and only sixty-one were discharged as 'incurable'.[31] It is not surprising that the volunteer physicians involved in this scheme wished their instructions to be followed dutifully by the patients and declined help to those who did not show a proper degree of respect for the physician and his prescription. Non-compliance could lead to disciplinary actions. The report for 1781 mentions, for example, that in the first six months five patients (out of 321) had been relegated 'because of their intemperance and wanton ruination of their bodies, their decided rebelliousness and coarse behavior toward their physicians, unmindful of all previous warnings'.[32]

In the second half of the eighteenth century physicians, health administrators, bureaucrats, philanthropists and magistrates, not only in Hanseatic towns but also in other German states, vigorously debated the advantages of visiting care over hospital treatment. Two of the most vociferous advocates of the superiority of outdoor medical relief, Senator Johann Arnold Günther[33] and Dr Daniel Nootnagel[34], came from Hamburg. Their preference for domiciliary medical aid rested on their experience first with the *Institut für Kranke Hausarme* and then with the 'Medicinal Deputation' of the *Armenanstalt* (General Poor Relief). The debate over which system offered more advantages even became the subject of an essay contest sponsored by the Royal Academy of Sciences in Göttingen in the 1790s.[35]

One of the most striking aspects of the poor relief reform in Hamburg in 1788 was its far-reaching and spiritedly pursued programme of providing free medical care even to non-registered poor, although here too there was a long list of precedents. Occasionally helping people of modest means and limited financial resources to pay for medical consultations and medication had long made up part of Christian and private charity. In its 'Instructions' to the poor relief officers, the *Armenanstalt* in Hamburg explained its medical relief programme as an attempt to extricate individuals and families from poverty and prevent others from sinking into destitution.[36] More investigation is required before it can be decided whether the various *Medizinalanstalten* which were founded about the same time in Bamberg, Detmold, Göttingen, Hannover, Oldenburg, Schwerin and other German towns were influenced by the Hamburg model of free medical care even for the non-registered poor. According to Mary Lindemann,[37] the unique programme of assistance for the so-called *nicht-eingezeichnete Arme*, was closely connected to the new perception of the labouring poor and of the important role they had come to play in Hamburg's growing economy at the end of the eighteenth century, which made it less likely for workers to be temporarily reduced to poverty.

The *Armenanstalt* in Hamburg offered a wide variety of medical assistance, including free treatment by physicians and surgeons, free medication, trusses and bandages, the help of a midwife in childbirth and a free stay in lying-in wards for poverty-stricken and unwed mothers[38] as well as special food allowances and even sick benefits that exceeded normal levels of support for paupers. Its scale of medical aid is indeed impressive, handling almost 50,000 cases from 1788 to 1801. Most interesting is the gradual extension of medical care to the non-registered poor, by which many members of the lower classes became eligible for free medical aid. The numbers of non-registered poor who applied for free medical care grew rapidly. In the beginning they constituted about 12 per cent of all patients. By 1799 there were 1,351 non-registered poor (i.e. 40 per cent) among those who received free medical assistance.[39] Caspar Voght, one of the fathers of poor relief reform in Hamburg, took pride in these impressive numbers, arguing that 'the increase of the non-registered poor treated among the sick shows how much this procedure contributes to the attainment of our goals of preventing destitution through timely assistance'.[40] To reduce expenses, the *Armenanstalt* instituted in 1793 a programme of 'half-free' medical care for those who could not afford to pay a physician's fee but were able to buy medicines if provided at the low rates set in the famous Hamburg 'Paupers Pharmacopoeia' of which three much acclaimed editions were published in the period 1781–1804.[41]

This medical relief programme thus extended to another project. In 1781 there was a decision to draw up a special pharmacopoeia for the poor, i.e. an authoritative list of the nature, quality and composition of drugs, which would function as a prescribing guide for local physicians involved in the medical relief programme. It was also supposed to provide a rule to which the apothecaries should adhere. The Hamburg magistrates also fixed the prices for these drugs. By controlling the price of drugs listed in the 'Paupers Pharmacopia' the *Armenanstalt* saved considerably on expenditure for medication.[42] Although the number of simple or composed drugs which officially could be administered to the poor was considerable, there can be no doubt that the poor patient got those remedies which according to contemporary pharmaceutical knowledge and standard therapeutics practice were supposed to provide an effective cure. And these drugs were not necessarily always the cheapest ones. There were, of course, many cheaper substitutes listed for many drugs (e.g. *oleum ricini, lignum quassiae – Bitterholz*) which can be found in prescriptions for the ordinary clientele, but if a physician to the poor or a medical officer thought that such a rather expensive drug as, for example, Peruvian bark (*cortex chinae*) had to be given to a sick pauper he was allowed to do so.[43]

The importance of medical assistance within the framework of poor relief can be measured by many yardsticks. Certainly there is some evidence to suggest that the sick poor were a little bit better off in Hamburg than, for instance, in Lübeck or Bremen. The only available measure is the share medical aid had in the budget of the *Armenanstalten* in those cities. It does not come as a surprise that the largest sums still went for aid to the domiciled poor in the forms of alms, clothing, fuel and bread. In Hamburg, for example, free medical care for the poor amounted to between 5.03 and 8.65 per cent of the total expenditures of the *Armenanstalt* in the last decade of the eighteenth century. In comparison to Hamburg, where between 2,300 and 3,900 families were on the dole, the *Armenanstalt* in Lübeck (re-organised in 1783) had at the same time far fewer people on the relief roll (500–600). The absolute numbers were, of course, lower, but there is almost no difference in terms of percentages of the total expenditure. In Lübeck 73 to 84 per cent of the annual budget went for regular allowances or pensions for poor householders, thus far outweighing costs for medical care, which ranged between 5 and 12 per cent in the years 1785–1800.[44]

HOSPITAL CARE

Most 'medical' institutions in early modern Hanseatic towns were poor relief establishments. Neither in Lübeck, Hamburg or Bremen did a single or even uniform institutional framework for the provision of medical care exist. Medical assistance was, in practice, provided where it was needed, whether in general or special hospitals[45] (asylums, infirmaries, leper houses, plague hospitals, etc.), orphanages,[46] houses of correction or workhouses.[47] In some of these institutions medical care for the poor was more or less effectively combined with the regulation of behaviour.

The Hamburg hospitals differed from the ones in Bremen in not being connected, even administratively, with the city's new outdoor relief scheme. Although essentially independent, their activities were nevertheless increasingly supervised by the Hamburg Senate, a more indirect method of centralised control. Another major difference is that in the case of Bremen it is easier to suppose a more significant role for such institutions in the care and treatment of the poor than it is in the case of Hamburg and Lübeck. Bremen's interest in institutionalised medical care for the poor became more pronounced during the seventeenth century, but was not new in the post-Reformation period.[48] Outdoor medical relief was not given up, but generally there was more resort to closed institutions (infirmary, asylum, workhouse, orphanage) whose purpose was both to provide medical care and to inculcate social discipline.[49] The *Armenhaus*[50] founded in Bremen in 1698 was such a multifunctional institution. The foundation charter stipulated:

> Fünftens aber alle andere hiesige notdürftige Armen (außer den Kranken) sollen ohne eintzige Unterscheid, absonderlich ob dieselben arbeiten können oder nicht, in dieß neu errichtete Armenhaus respektive an- und aufgenommen, eingewiesen, eingeführet und notdürftiglich besorget werden, doch solcher Gestallt, daß diejenigen, welche Leibes-Constitution zur Arbeit geschickt, dazu auch angehalten werden, welche aber dazu unbequem, davon befreiet werden.[51]

The sick but not disabled poor, however, were sent to the local infirmary established in the quarter called the *Neustadt* in the early 1690s. In the first decades of its existence, the *Armenhaus* provided indoor relief for about 300 inmates. The pivotal role of the *Armenhaus* within the institutional framework of poor relief in Bremen becomes clear if one looks at the various responsibilities of its general manager. He was not only in charge of the inmates of the *Armenhaus*, he also supervised the monthly pensions paid to the poor on the relief roll (*Bucharme*), arranged burials for the poor, distributed alms to foreigners, and paid out special allowances for the sick poor. And last, but not least, he was partly responsible for operating the infirmary, the orphanage (*Blaues Waisenhaus*), and the local workhouse (*Zucht- und Arbeitshaus*).[52] We can see a very similar development in the case of Lübeck, where in 1601 the former monastery of St Anna was turned into a general poor relief agency, to which later on several other welfare institutions were added: a house of correction (1612), an infirmary (1643) and a workhouse (1778).[53] In the early nineteenth century the *St Annen Armen- und Werkhaus* provided indoor relief for about a thousand people per year, of which 80 to 90 per cent were in need of medical care.[54]

The Reformation not only seriously affected the practice of alms-giving, but also the way indoor relief was organised in most north German cities. Bremen, however, proved to be a special case because of the religious strife between Lutherans and Calvinists. The development of Reformed or more radical Protestantism in the second half of the sixteenth century, came to dominate also the organisation of poor relief in this city. By the 1680s the Lutheran leaders who were concerned about religious discrimination and doctrinal purity felt the need to establish their own poor relief institutions.[55] In 1691 they founded an orphanage for Lutheran children in order to preserve the rights of the *reine unveränderte Augsburgische Confession* [56] and even tried to get the parish relief back into their hands. From the late seventeenth- to the middle of the eighteenth century, religious strife continued to hamper the administration and centralisation of poor relief in this Hanseatic town. The neighbouring cities of Hamburg and Lübeck, however, were spared such detrimental confessionalism because they remained firmly Lutheran throughout the period under study in this chapter.

The majority of hospitals in Lübeck, Hamburg and Bremen were small, multi-purposed institutions, better prepared for the exigencies of poverty than of disease. The best known and longest-lived of these well endowed late medieval institutions are the *Heilig-Geist-Spitäler* in Hamburg[57] (first mentioned in 1247) and Lübeck[58] (founded in the thirteenth century). Since the first half of the seventeenth century the hospital of the Holy Spirit in Hamburg had a surgeon on stipend. The first university-trained physician does not appear in the payrolls before 1731. The main purpose of this hospital was to care for those who, because of old age or chronic illnesses, depended on institutional relief. Occasionally the hospital administrators covered the cost for an expensive cure of one of the inmates. In 1602, for example, the hospital of the Holy Spirit paid the expenses for two blind inmates who underwent an eye operation (*Starstich*).[59] In 1632 Master Jonas, the hospital surgeon, was given the large sum of thirty-six marks to attend a poor woman suffering from an unknown ailment.[60] The usually tiny fraction of its expenditure which went on drugs and medicines underlines, however, the subordinate role this type of hospital played in the provision of medical relief for the poor. The account book of 1634, for example, mentions sundry expenses for *allerhand getihtilliertes Wasser, Brusttrüncke und derogleichen für die kranken Armen*.[61] Diet in these hospitals was rather a means of sustenance than part of a therapeutic strategy; special food for the sick is also sometimes mentioned in the account books. The food which the hospitalised poor, whether sick or not, could expect in those general hospitals was plentiful enough to feed any able-bodied person and was normally of better quality than they might hope to enjoy in the outside world.[62]

Other hospitals performed a number of functions for the inmates and for the city. The *Pesthof*[63] and the *Hiobshospital*[64] in Hamburg, for example, were first used by the city in the case of infectious diseases but later on for the treatment of other types of disease as well. The Hamburg authorities were plainly more concerned about the 'French disease' than, for example, the magistrates in Lübeck or Bremen, which did not establish a special hospital for the treatment of paupers suffering from the 'Pox'. About 30 per cent of the patients of the Hamburg *Hiobshospital* had been referred to this *lazarhouse* from other welfare institutions (workhouse, orphanage, general hospital, etc.).[65] A cure lasted usually between five to twelve weeks. The daily ration amounted to two shillings in 1681.[66] In the beginning the hospital administrators arranged a contract for one patient for twelve marks then eighteen marks (1625). Paid at first on the usual contract basis, the barber-surgeon employed by the *Hiobshospital* later on received a lump sum or stipend amouting to sixty marks per annum. During the Thirty Years' War and the second half of the eighteenth century the number of patients treated per year ranged between fifty and one hundred.[67] A comparison of expenditures on drugs and medicines in various types of hospitals reveals that expenses for medical assistance normally accounted for less than 4 per cent of the total expenditure.[68] In the *Hiobshospital* in Hamburg, as in similar hospitals specialising in the treatment of syphilitics, these expenses ranged between 5 to 20 per cent of the total expenditure in the years 1670–1800.[69] There can be no doubt that the higher expenses on drugs and fees for physicians and barber-surgeons in those special hospitals indicate a new quality and intensity of medical care (not only for the poor!) which later on becomes the characteristic feature of the modern clinic.

In contrast to the general hospitals in early modern Hamburg, Bremen and Lübeck, which cared for a varied clientele (the aged, the infirm, the disabled, the unwanted child, the pilgrim, the itinerant worker, the temporary or seasonal migrant), these three Hanseatic towns prided themselves on some institutions which might be called infirmaries rather than hospitals in the traditional sense of the word. This label can, for instance, be applied to the *Gast- und Krankenhaus*[70] in Hamburg during the sixteenth century, to the *Krankenhaus* affiliated with the *Armenanstalt* in Bremen[71] established in the 1680s and the famous *Pesthof*[72] in Hamburg, which despite its name very soon ceased to be a hospital used only in times of plague, and also it kept its quarantine function until the early eighteenth century. By the 1750s the *Pesthof* admitted around 1,100 in-patients a year, which represented a fourfold increase since the 1660s.[73] These figures suggest that a sizeable proportion of Hamburg's poor came in contact with institutional medical care at some point of their lifetime. The admission policy mirrors the fact that this hospital was not yet dominated by its surgeons and physicians. Unlike so many other hospitals which became proto-clinics (Michel Foucault) in the eighteenth century, the *Pesthof* managed with a very small medical personel until the beginning of the nineteenth century. By the last decades of the Ancien Régime, the *Pesthof*, which was already known as *Krankenhof*, had a surgeon plus assistants on stipend and a doctor who visited the hospital three times a week and remained on call as well. It does not come as a surprise that in the middle of the eighteenth century the average length of stay was three years. In 1756 for example, the hospital had 954 inmates at the end of the year. During the following year 533 were newly admitted, 344 (23 per cent) died and 162 were discharged as cured.[74] According to the admission rolls of this hospital, recovery from scabies, phtisis and various leg ailments involved long-term treatment. Such attendance could last weeks or even months, and prove costly. For a poor patient, the *Pesthof* and similar institutions, labelled infirmaries by contemporary writers, offered accommodation, a fairly good diet, medical care and few responsibilities save some form of gratitude (e.g. prayers). There can be no doubt that the older conceptions of a hospital's social functions died hard and that patients as well as poor relief administrators in Hamburg and elsewhere tried to use these institutions to provide care as well as cure up to the early nineteenth century.

CONCLUSION

By the early seventeenth century, the magistrates of Bremen, Lübeck and Hamburg had evolved a range of expedients and institutions to deal with the sick poor. Those institutions represent an attempt to provide cost-effective short-term medical treatment and supervision for the sick but potentially able poor, in most cases on a joint basis with other central poor relief agencies and the parishes but with the main responsibility resting on the city magistrates. For the local authorities, there were obvious adavantages of flexibility in the connexions of hospitals and infirmaries with the specific functions of the deacons in the parishes, workhouses, orphanages and other welfare institutions, and with other relevant practices supervised by the municipality, such as apprenticeship and medical relief programmes. This comparison of various health care institutions and outdoor medical relief in three Hanseatic towns suggests that medical care was a significant component of early modern welfare provision.

Even institutionally there was a degree of long-term continuity in the medical relief system of some of these cities. In the sixteenth- and seventeenth century, the *Pesthof* in Hamburg was an isolation hospital and then developed gradually into an 'infirmary'. In 1797 it also changed its name to a more appropiate one: *Krankenhof*. At the beginning of the twentieth century the *Armenhaus* in Bremen (founded in 1698) served as an old age home. The famous *Heiligen-Geist-Spital* in Lübeck with its imposing architectural structure had changed from hospital to an old-age home, and finally to a museum, the second being, as can be easily noticed, not so far from the first as we nowadays might imagine.

NOTES

1 On Hyperius' importance as a poor relief reformer, see Robert Jütte, 'Andreas Hyperius (1511–64) und die Reform des frühneuzeitlichen Armenwesens', *Archiv für Reformationsgeschichte*, 75 (1984), 113–138.

2 Andreas Hyperius, *The Regiment of the Povertie*, London 1572, f. 10v.

3 Cf. Gerhard Kaberlah, 'Der soziale Gedanke in Bugenhagens Braunschweiger Kirchenordnung', *Jahrbuch der Gesellschaft für niedersächsische Kirchengeschichte*, 51 (1953), 113–17; Frank Peter Lane, *Poverty and Poor Relief in the German Church Orders of Johann Bugenhagen, 1485–1558*, doctoral dissertation, Ohio State University 1973; Ursula Rotzoll, 'Kastenordnungen der Reformationszeit. Von der mittelalterlichen zur neuzeitlichen Armenpflege', unpublished

thesis, University of Marburg 1969. See also Chapter 2 of this volume.

4 On the Reformation in Hamburg in general, see Rainer Postel, *Die Reformation in Hamburg 1517–28*, Gütersloh 1986. For a detailed discussion of the poor relief reform in Hamburg in the late 1520s, see Rotzoll, *Kastenordnungen*, 54 ff.

5 'Gottes-Kasten-Ordnung. Anfang der Kisten / so tho Underholdinghe der Armen in Sunte Nicolaus Kercken binnen Hamborch gestellet is', 16 August 1527, in Nicolaus Staphorst, *Historia Ecclesiae Hamburgensis diplomatica*, Hamburg 1723–29, part 1, vol. 2, 112–23.

6 English translation by Mary Lindemann, *Patriots and Paupers. Hamburg 1712–1830*, New York 1990, 15–16.

7 Emil Sehling (ed.) *Die Evangelischen Kirchenordnungen des XVI. Jahrhunderts*, Leipzig 1913, vol. 5, 534.

8 Sehling, *Kirchenordnungen*, 361.

9 Cf. Carter Lindberg, 'There should be no beggars among Christians: Karlstadt, Luther and the origins of poor relief', *Church History*, 46 (1977), 313–34. See also Chapter 2 of this volume.

10 Johannes Böckel, *Pestordnung der Stadt Hamburch*, Hamburg 1597, 23. Cf. also Lindemann, *Patriots*, 227, note 50.

11 Quoted in Lindemann, *Patriots*, 103.

12 Cf. Robert Jütte, *Poverty and Deviance in Early Modern Europe*, Cambridge 1994, 41.

13 Quoted by Lindemann, *Patriots*, 103.

14 See Norbert Finzsch, *Obrigkeiten und Unterschichten. Zur Geschichte der rheinischen Unterschichten gegen Ende des 18. und zu Beginn des 19. Jahrhunderts*, Stuttgart 1990, 306.

15 Cf. Ortwin Pelc, 'Die Armenversorgung in Lübeck in der Ersten Hälfte des 19. Jahrhunderts', *Zeitschrift des Vereins für Lübeckische Geschichte*, 66 (1986), 143–84, especially 173. On the housing conditions of the poor in north German towns, see Jürgen Ellermeyer, 'Grundeigentum, Arbeits- und Wohnverhältnisse. Bemerkungen zur Sozialgeschichte spätmittelalterlich-frühneuzeitlicher Städte', *Lübecker Schriften zur Archäologie und Kunstgeschichte*, 4 (1980), 71–95; the same: 'Die Armenanstalt und die Wohnungsnot Ende des 18. Jahrhunderts: Mit Schwung in die Krise (1788–95)', in Erich Braun and Franklin Kopitzsch (eds) *Zwangsläufig oder abwendbar? 200 Jahre Hamburgisch Allgemeine Armenanstalt*, Hamburg, 1990, 46–96; Klaus Schwarz, 'Der Bremer Wohnungsmarkt um die Mitte des 18. Jahrhunderts', *Vierteljahrschrift für Sozial- und Wirtschaftsgeschichte*, 55 (1968), 193–213.

16 Lindemann, *Patriots*, 107.

17 On this Church Order which was drawn up by Johann Timmann but heavily influenced by Bugenhagen's ideas, cf. R. Feuss, *Kurz gefasste Geschichte der Armenpflege, die künftige Armenfürsorge und die Einrichung eines Wohlfahrtsamtes*, Bremen 1919, 7; M. J. Funk, *Geschichte und Statistik des Bremischen Armenwesens*, Bremen 1913, 1; W. von Bippen, 'Ausbildung der Bürgerlichen Armenpflege in Bremen', *Bremisches Jahrbuch*, 11 (1880), 143–61, especially 145; Franziskus Petri, *Unser*

Lieben Frauen Diakonie. 400 Jahre evangelischer Liebestätigkeit in Bremen, Bremen 1925, 21.

18   Cf. Petri, *Diakonie*, 40.

19   Cf. Lindemann, *Patriots*, 107.

20   Cf. Petri, *Diakonie*, 71.

21   Cf. Petri, *Diakonie*, 60.

22   In Bremen, for instance, the late sixteenth-century account books of the *Armenkasten* seldom refer expressly to special payments for the sick; cf. Petri, *Diakonie*, 33.

23   Cf. Petri, *Diakonie*, 32, note 2.

24   Cf. Petri, *Diakonie*, 78.

25   On this office, see Arthur W. Russell (ed.) *The Town and the State Physician in Europe from the Middle Ages to the Enlightenment*, Wiesbaden 1981.

26   Cf. Petri, *Diakonie*, 61.

27   The free medical treatment of the needy has become a topos in medical history; but social reality and ethical obligations were often two different pairs of shoes; cf. J. H. Donhoff, *Der Arzt und sein Honorar im Wandel der Zeit*, Zurich 1968.

28   Cf. Hansjörg Reupke, *Zur Geschichte der Ausübung der Heilkunde durch nichtapprobierte Personen in Hamburg von den Anfänge bis zum Erlass des 'Heilpraktikergesetzes' im Jahre 1939*, Herzogenrath 1978, 46.

29   Cf. Lindemann, *Patriots*, 103; Almuth Weidmann, *Die Arzneiversorgung der Armen zu Beginn der Industrialisierung im deutschen Sprachgebiet, besonders in Hamburg*, Braunschweig 1982, 21.

30   Quoted in Lindemann, *Patriots*, 104.

31   Figures according to Weidmann, *Arzneiversorgung*, 24.

32   Quoted in Lindemann, *Patriots*, 105.

33   Johann Arnold Günther, *Über die Einrichtung der mit der Hamburgischen Allgemeinen Armenanstalt verbundenen Kranken-Besuchs-Anstalt*, Leipzig 1793.

34   Daniel Nootnagell, 'Über Krankenanstalten', *Hamburgische Address-Comtoir-Nachrichten*, no. 23, 1785, 177–9, no. 24, 1785, 185–7. Cf. also Gunnar Holst, 'Zur Geschichte des Armenarztwesens der Stadt Hamburg, 1713–1921', medical dissertation, University of Aachen 1987, 36–7.

35   Cf. Lindemann, *Patriots*, 261, note 23.

36   Cf. Lindemann, 'The Allgemeine Armenanstalt and the Non-Registered Poor', in Franklin Kopitzsch (ed.) *Zwangsläufig oder abwendbar? 200 Jahre Hamburgische Allgemeine Armenanstalt. Symposium der Patriotischen Gesellschaft von 1765*, Hamburg 1990, 37–45, especially 42.

37   Cf. Lindemann, *Armenanstalt*, 38. See also M.Lindemann, 'Urban Growth and Medical Care. Hamburg, 1788–1815', in J. Barry and C. Jones (eds), *Medicine and Charity before the Welfare State*, London 1991, 113–32.

38   Cf. Mary Lindemann, 'Fürsorge für arme Wöchnerinnen in Hamburg um 1800: die Beschreibung eines "Entbindungs-Winkels" ', *Gesnerus*, 39 (1982), 395–403. See also her article 'Maternal Politics: the

principles and practice of maternity care in eighteenth-century Hamburg', *Journal of Family History*, 9 (1984), 44–63.

39 Cf. Lindemann, *Patriots*, 170.
40 Quoted in Lindemann, *Patriots*, 170.
41 Cf. Weidmann, *Arzneiversorgung*, 108–10.
42 Cf. Weidmann, *Arzneiversorgung*, 45–6.
43 See Weidmann, *Arzneiversorgung*, 144–6.
44 Pelc, *Armenanstalt*, 116.
45 On the major hospitals in these three Hanseatic towns, see for instance Dieter Boedecker, 'Die Entwicklung der hamburgischen Hospitäler seit der Gründung der Stadt bis 1800 aus ärztlicher Sicht', medical dissertation, University of Hamburg 1974; Wilhelm Stier, *Das Heiligen-Geist-Hospital in Lübeck*, Lübeck 1961; Wilhelm Plessing, *Das Heilige-Geist-Hospital in Lübeck im 17. und 18. Jahrhundert*, Lübeck 1914; Dörte Stolle, 'Das Heiligen Geist Hospital zu Lübeck. Eine historisch-sozialhygienische Studie', medical dissertation, Lübeck 1970; Walter Hayessen, 'Die Gebäude der Lübecker Wohlfahrtspflege', doctoral dissertation, TH Braunschweig 1925; Wilhelm Arnold Walte, *Dieser Stat Armenhaus zum Behten und Arbeyten. Geschichte des Armenhauses zu Bremen 1698–1866 mit weiteren Beiträgen zur bremischen Sozialgeschichte*, ed. Peter Galperin, Frankfurt am Main 1979, 241–68.
46 On orphanages, see Gerhard Commichau, 'Zur Geschichte der hamburgischen Jugendfürsorge im 18. Jahrhundert', doctoral dissertation, Hamburg 1961; Meno Günther Kiehn, *Das Hamburger Waisenhaus. Geschichtlich beschreibend dargestellt*, Hamburg 1821; B. A. J. Vogelsang, *Das Hamburger Waisenhaus. Geschichtlich beschreibend dargestellt von 1597 bis auf die neuere Zeit*, Hamburg 1889; Charles Hornung Petit, *Das Lübecker Waisenhaus*, Lübeck 1918.
47 See, for example, Kai Detlev Sievers, *Leben in Armut. Zeugnisse der Armutskultur aus Lübeck und Schleswig-Holstein vom Mittelalter bis ins 20. Jahrhundert*, Heide 1991, 67–72; Robert von Hippel, 'Beiträge zur Geschichte der Freiheitsstrafe', *Zeitschrift für die gesamte Strafrechtswissenschaft*, 18 (1898), 419–94, 608–66 (on Lübeck: 620–30); A. Behrend and I. Koepsel, 'Zur Geschichte des Bremer Gefängniswesens unter besonderer Berücksichtigung des Beschäftigungssystems', unpublished thesis, University of Bremen 1979; Adolf Streng, *Geschichte der Gefängnisverwaltung in Hamburg 1622–1872*, Hamburg 1890; Heinrich Sieveking, 'Hamburger Gefängnisfürsorge im 18. Jahrhundert', *Altonaische Zeitschrift*, 3 (1933–4), 94–106.
48 See Petri, *Diakonie*, 121, 126.
49 On the concept of social discipline in poor relief, see Robert Jütte, 'Poor Relief and Social Discipline in Early Modern Europe', *European Studies Review*, 11 (1981), 25–52; Martin Dinges, 'Frühneuzeitliche Armenfürsorge als Sozialdisziplinierung? Probleme mit einem Konzept', *Geschichte und Gesellschaft*, 17 (1991), 5–29. Cf. also my rejoinder, ' "Disziplin zu predigen ist eine Sache, sich ihr zu unterwerfen eine andere" (Cervantes) – Prolegomena zu einer

Sozialgeschichte der Armut diesseits und jenseits des Fortschritts', *Geschichte und Gesellschaft*, 17 (1991), 92–111.

50 On the history of this centralised poor relief institution, see Walte, *Armenhaus*.

51 Reprinted in Walte, *Armenhaus*, 282–3

52 Cf. Petri, *Diakonie*, 143.

53 Cf. Robert von Hippel, 'Zur Geschichte des Werk- und Zuchthauses zu St Annen', *Mitteilungen des Vereins für Lübeckische Geschichte und Altertumskunde*, 8 (1897–8), 146–58; Friedrich Bruns, 'Zur Geschichte des St Annen-Klosters', *Zeitschrift des Vereins für Lübeckische Geschichte und Altertumskunde*, 17 (1915), 173–204.

54 Pelc, 'Armenfürsorge', 147.

55 On this special battlefield of seventeenth-century confessionalism in Bremen, see Feuss, *Geschichte*, 9; Bippen, 'Ausbildung', 150–2; Otto Veeck, *Geschichte der Reformierten Kirche in Bremen*, Bremen 1909, 215–16.

56 Quoted in Bippen, 'Ausbildung', 150.

57 On the history of this hospital, see Boedecker, *Entwicklung*, 64–111; C. F. Gaedechens, 'Geschichte des Hospitals zum heiligen Geist in Hamburg', *Zeitschrift des Vereins für Hamburgische Geschichte*, 8 (1889), 343–420.

58 Cf. Bernhard Schlippe, 'Das Heiligen-Geist-Hospital zu Lübeck. Eine baugeschichtliche Betrachtung mittelalterlichen Hospitalwesens', *Der Wagen*, 1963, 23–30.

59 Cf. Boedecker, *Entwicklung*, 92.

60 Cf. Boedecker, *Entwicklung*, 88.

61 Quoted in Boedeker, *Entwicklung*, 90.

62 Cf. Robert Jütte, 'Diets in Welfare Institutions and in Outdoor Poor Relief in Early Modern Western Europe', *Ethnologia Europaea*, 16 (1987), 117–35.

63 Cf. Boedecker, *Entwicklung*, 229–326.

64 Cf. Helmut Puff, 'Jobst von Overbeck (1663–1726) und das Hamburger Hiobshospital', thesis, University of Hamburg 1987.

65 See Boedecker, *Entwicklung*, 196.

66 Cf. Boedecker, *Entwicklung*, 211.

67 Boedecker, *Entwicklung*, 189, 224, table 2, appendix.

68 Cf. Colin Jones, *Charity and Bienfaisance. The treatment of the poor in the Montpellier Region, 1740–1815*, Cambridge 1982, 122, table 10; Robert Jütte, 'Syphilis and Confinement: Hospitals in early modern Germany', in Norbert Finzsch and Robert Jütte (eds) *Institutions of Confinement*, New York 1996, 97–116.

69 See Boedecker, *Entwicklung*, 210, table 1.

70 Cf. Boedecker, *Entwicklung*, 112–63.

71 See Petri, *Diakonie*, 113, 127, 145.

72 Cf. Boedecker, *Entwicklung*, 229–326.

73 Cf. Boedecker, *Entwicklung*, 323.

74 See Boedecker, *Entwicklung*, 297.

Chapter 6

Poor relief and health care provision in sixteenth-century Denmark

Thomas Riis

A major question concerning sixteenth-century poor relief in Northern Europe is to know to what extent the Reformation changed existing forms of assistance, suppressing or modifying them or introducing new ones. The first thing we need to know is: who were the poor?

According to the Danish Carmelite friar Poul Helgesen, writing in 1528, there were three major causes of poverty: calamities, idleness and carelessness. He recognised that some people were poor because they had been born in distress and did not know how to improve their condition; interestingly enough, he regarded idleness as well as industry as dispositions granted by God. In other cases, Helgesen wrote, poverty was caused by adversities or by vice. As a matter of principle, the community should assist its members when necessary, but wealthy persons ought to take care of their poor relatives.[1]

That victims of calamities – fire, shipwreck, captivity, loss of a husband or a parent – deserved aid, was recognised by the Reformers as well as by their medieval predecessors. This group of poor was fairly easy to identify, and in the local community people would know the cause of their misfortune. It was much more difficult to ascertain whether or not the able-bodied poor did not work because of idleness or because they could find no work.

Most late medieval and early modern writers did not recognise the problem of underemployment, but considered the able-bodied poor as simply lazy. Actually, a new attitude towards work had developed during the fourteenth century and was taken over by the subsequent periods. In late medieval thought, the principal aim of work was to earn one's daily bread, but work was also considered a remedy against idleness and concupiscence. In the Italian preacher

Simone Fidati di Cascia (d. 1348) we find a representative of the latter view; according to him work was so salutary that a rich man who had no need to work ought nevertheless to do so and give the money earned to the poor.[2]

No wonder then, if in times of crisis work was considered a civic duty. The Swedish urban statute from about 1350 obliged every able-bodied adult to work, unless their fortune allowed them to live for a year. England introduced similar acts in 1349 and again two years later compelling every able-bodied person under sixty to work. Analogous rules were enacted in Castile in 1351 and in Portugal in 1375.[3] Most of these statutes were passed shortly after the Black Death, reflecting its consequences in the decline of the working population. That this was a major concern is further confirmed by a Danish statute passed in 1354, which limited the use of capital punishment and maiming because of the shortage of population.[4]

We all know the classical medieval justification of begging: the almsgiver helps the poor person who in return prays for the giver's soul. Besides the individual gift, private charities were established.[5] However, the system was not flawless and abuse did occur. We know that allegedly poor inmates of the houses of the Holy Spirit were active in trade and not every beggar could be considered needy.[6] Franciscan, Dominican, and Carmelite friars went begging, and many others too. Thus regulation was needed: Christian II's legislation of 1522 tried to solve the problem.

As a matter of principle begging was reserved to Franciscans, Carmelites and Dominicans and priests belonging to the houses of the Holy Spirit following the Order of St Augustine. Monasteries with landed property could only collect alms with permission from the king;[7] moreover, begging was allowed on behalf of lepers.[8]

It is interesting that the articles try to restrict begging by defining a category of 'deserving poor'. Able-bodied beggars should be expelled, unless they were ready to work. The right to beg was restricted to the sick, the poor and to cripples unable to earn their living themselves. Each month the town government should control them and give them a badge as proof of their authorisation to collect alms.[9] The obligation to work thus appeared for the first time in Denmark, even if it had to wait until 1537 before it was legally established.[10]

The number of non-deserving beggars appears to have considerably increased towards the end of the Middle Ages, thus the need for a distinction between able-bodied and deserving poor made itself ever more felt. The late medieval statutes on beggars issued by German towns made the distinction; Luther made it in 1520,[11] and the Danish government two years later. But where the obligation to work had initially been an economic measure to remedy the lack of manpower, in the sixteenth- and seventeenth centuries it was advocated for moral as well as for economic reasons; for mercantilist economics un- and under-employment was a waste of resources.[12] Danish social policy after 1520 followed this international current.

At the same time the abolition through the Reformation of most Catholic holidays meant that the working week increased by 15 to 20 per cent, at any rate in towns. Thus if the quantity of work remained constant, there would be less work left for the individual, with underemployment as a consequence.

No wonder, then, if the number of able-bodied poor increased, seeing their only source of income in begging. The statute of 1536 had allowed places in hospitals to the weakest among the deserving poor, while the rest were allowed to collect alms in the traditional way; however, able-bodied beggars were to suffer capital punishment. These harsh rules were modified in the following year: the deserving poor born in town were to be authorised to beg, the able-bodied poor were to be offered work or expelled if they would not work,[13] but – what to do if there was no work to be had?

Obviously, it proved impossible to have these new rules respected which corresponded to economic reality in only such a limited way.[14] Because the collection of alms was only authorised in one's parish of origin, non-natives were expelled, thus swelling the group of vagrants in quest of income somewhere else. The government saw to it that criminal elements were punished,[15] but apparently closed its eyes to illegal alms-giving.[16] Gypsies were, however, to be banned from Denmark.[17]

The statute of 1558 art. 62 repeated Christian II's legislation on beggars in all essential respects,[18] but apparently the rules were not observed; the numerous repetitions of the legislation demonstrate this clearly.[19] In 1576 the government ordered local authorities to arrest idle men and to send them to Copenhagen,[20] but six years later it had to recognise that in some parishes the number of beggars had increased so much that even the native, deserving poor could not be supported.[21] After some years of preparations, a new statute was promulgated on 27 December 1587. On all essential points it remained faithful to the principles expressed in Christian II's legislation, but refined and developed the mechanisms of control.[22]

How had late medieval charity been financed? First, we know of the existence of a multitude of pious foundations with the aim of relieving poverty, at least temporarily, through distributions of food and drink. Very often they were connected with a votive mass in memory of the founder. Thus in about 1175 the abbot of Æbelholt made the disposition that on the anniversary of his death a mass should be held, special fare should be served to the monks of his monastery, and twelve poor persons should receive a meal on that day.[23] Or one could mention the dwellings for the poor such as those constructed by the councillor Mogens Steen at Køge in 1523.[24] Besides these two types of medieval charity – the chantry and the endowment – private or institutional almsgiving should not be underestimated. The rural monasteries with their extensive landed property were able to spend important sums on alms, and this practice continued for a long time after the Reformation. In 1552 the prior of Antvorskov (secularised in 1580) complained that travellers used the monastery as a hostel, following pre-Reformation tradition; the monastery of Ringsted (secularised in 1592) provided in 1576–7 twenty to thirty meals a week to poor persons, and as late as 1641–4 the school of Sorø (as a monastery secularised in 1580) was giving food to between 600 and 1,100 persons a year.

In the numerous cases where a landed monastery was not replaced by another institution like the schools of Sorø or Herlufsholm, the charitable distributions ceased when the monastery was secularised; in general, its property was added to the demesne, or the whole estate with the buildings was sold to members of the aristocracy.[25]

The urban convents of the mendicant orders had in many cases been dissolved before the definitive victory of Luther's ideas with the victory of the Reformation in Denmark in 1536. Often the buildings were ceded to the town government to use as a hospital for the poor.[26] However, the mendicant orders in Denmark had been reformed a short time before the Reformation – from 1517 all Franciscans were Observants – and consequently had little landed property, often only the buildings and the plots they stood on. Although the constructions were solid and often in good repair, supplementary income had to be found if they were to accomodate a number of poor without recourse to begging. The introduction of poor rates might have been a logical consequence after the

Reformation, but for some reason this was only attempted in about 1630, and then only in a few towns.

The abolition of the chantries might have furnished this source of revenue, but in several cases the land reverted to the descendants of the founders if they could prove that it had been given by their ancestors for the celebration of masses. This rule, however, only applied to members of the aristocracy, and only if the donations were not to benefit the poor and sick.[27] Thus the government took care in protecting the interests of the hospitals of the Holy Spirit in particular. Further, we should not exaggerate the importance of the Danish chantries: often the endowment consisted only of a farm ceded in return for the annual celebration of a votive mass.[28] Foundations of altars would on the other hand be much richer, more spectacular, and far fewer.[29] So much remains hypothetical in this area, but in another field – health care provisions and hospitals – the sources do allow us to see what happened as a consequence of the Reformation.

HOSPITALS

Although experienced private healers must have existed in medieval Denmark, for example women who had often assisted others in childbirth, medical expertise was almost exclusively to be found in the monasteries; excavations at the Cistercian monastery of Cara Insula in Central Jutland and at Augustinian Æbelholt in North Zealand have yielded much information on the history of diseases and medicine in medieval Denmark.[30] Most convents and monasteries were, however, closed at the Reformation;[31] despite the fact that a limited number continued for a generation or two after the official abolition of the Catholic rite, the monastic hospitals ceased to exist when the monasteries were closed. This happened in 1560 at both Cara Insula and Æbelholt.[32]

Besides these institutions, hospitals for lepers cared for the sick, while the houses of the Holy Spirit appear to have cared for the poor as well.

The isolation of lepers in hospitals may have proved effective: in 1542 the government noticed that leprosy was gradually disappearing; consequently, leper hospitals could be merged with other hospitals. The surviving lepers should be moved to the general hospitals, where special houses for them were to be constructed. Thus their isolation should be maintained even if the hospitals united,[33] and this must be seen as an attempt at improving management in the domain of disease.

The union of hospitals was a measure introduced a long time before the Reformation. King Christian I (1448–81) had already granted St George's Hospital with St John's Chapel outside Randers to the convent of the order of St Bridget at Mariager;[34] and at Aalborg, the Holy Spirit Hospital undertook in 1513 to admit lepers, because the leper hospital dedicated to St George had been united with it.[35] Moreover, at Copenhagen, St George's leper hospital had been granted in 1517 to the Carmelites of Elsinore, who were to run it as a hospital for the poor and sick.[36] After the Reformation St George's hospital, in which some patients were still living, was transferred to the capital's Holy Spirit Hospital. It may be tempting to explain the incorporation of leper hospitals by the gradual disappearance of the disease, and to consider the unification of leper hospitals as a purely administrative measure introduced when appropriate, and not one generated by the Protestant reformers.

Leper hospitals often owned land, which was generally cultivated by copyholders paying rent to the institutions. Another source of income was the payment in kind by the peasants of certain localities (*herreder*); in return the hospital was to admit lepers from these districts. This type of arrangement is known from Ribe, Copenhagen and Næstved in 1523,[37] from Slagelse in 1530 and 1541,[38] as well as from Aarhus in 1541. Only for St Catherine's leper hospital at Aarhus are further particulars known: each peasant from seven *herreder* around Aarhus was to give three bushels of grain to the hospital every year.[39] Besides these revenues from agriculture, alms most likely continued to play an important role in the leper hospitals' economy. Christian II's legislative initiatives, which in many respects were taken up again after the Reformation, tried to limit begging. However, in towns with lepers, one or two persons were allowed to beg at the town gates on behalf of the lepers.[40] Similar arrangements were made in the rural districts.[41]

The other type of hospital which survived the Reformation was the Holy Spirit Hospital. About twenty-eight such institutions are known; their main functions were to care for the poor as well as for the sick. The hospitals and houses of the Order of the Holy Spirit (unlike their convents) did not belong to it despite their dedication, even if in a few towns – Aalborg, Copenhagen, Malmø, Nakskov and Randers – a Holy Spirit House was transformed into a monastery of the Order.[42] The revenues came mainly from land and almsgiving; thus in 1493 the Pope authorised the Malmø monastery to collect alms in the diocese of Lund as well as on the island of Gotland.[43] Although the Reformation at Malmø abolished the monasteries – the Holy Spirit was to be a town hall and the Franciscan monastery was to be a hospital for the sick and poor[44] – begging remained an important source of income for the new Lutheran hospital,[45] which was allowed to take over land belonging to the chantries.[46]

Besides the Protestant government's ambition to eliminate possible centres of resistance to the new faith,[47] economic motives were certainly also important for the merging of hospitals after the Reformation. Real estate was obviously an important source of revenue and so also, after the Reformation, were tithes, as many charitable institutions were granted the royal part of the tithes of certain parishes. Thus the royal tithes of thirty-nine parishes were assigned to the hospital of Copenhagen in 1555, which was to provide two meals a day to twenty poor and industrious students,[48] and in 1549, the peasants of Funen, Langeland, and Taasinge were requested to hand over their tithes of cattle for the benefit of the hospital in Odense.[49]

The abolition of the chantries rendered it sometimes possible to increase a hospital's real estate, as a case from Næstved shows. A certain Laurits Persen of Tyvelse took legal action against the parson of St Peter's in Næstved over a chantry endowed by Laurits Persen's late uncle. The plaintiff maintained that the services, in return for which the real estate had been given, were no longer held, but the clergyman offered services according to the Church Ordinance. Protestant services instead of Catholic mass would, of course, not promise salvation for the founder's soul, so in the end a compromise was found. According to the text of the endowment, the heirs could transfer it to other divine services, if the mass was no longer celebrated; the parties agreed to give the endowed house to the poor and sick in the Holy Spirit House of Næstved.[50]

Despite such measures, institutionalised poor relief could not manage without alms. A royal letter of 22 April 1517 authorised a certain Hans Tysk at Skagen to build a house and chapel outside town, to let sick persons live there and to receive alms collected for their maintenance.[51] In 1532 the Lutheran parson of Trelleborg was allowed to collect alms for the local hospital in every *herred*, and in the same year the sick and poor (i.e. the hospital) of Køge were granted the right of alms-collecting in four *herreder* around the town.[52] According to a royal letter of 1536, Copenhagen hospital could collect alms in the diocese of Zealand;[53] in 1552 and 1557 the hospitals of Aarhus and Næstved obtained similar permissions,[54] and four years later the hospital of the capital was again allowed to collect alms in Zealand. Perhaps it had tried to make ends meet without alms from outside Copenhagen, but had had to give up because of the increasing number of people in need.[55] In 1562 the Scanian school pupils were allowed to beg in certain *herreder*, because alms from the towns were insufficient,[56] and Varberg hospital was granted the royal part of the tithes of one *herred*, as its only source of income until then had been alms.[57]

Occasionally the sources mention the planned number of occupants in the hospitals, which, we should remember, often remained dwellings for the elderly rather than infirmaries. When the Carmelite friars of Elsinore were allowed to build a hospital in 1516 (one dedicated to the sick) for sick foreign mariners, it was to have eight to ten beds.[58] In 1532 the hospital of Nykøbing Falster could accommodate five persons as residents with board and lodging, four more apparently had to provide their own meals;[59] at Nakskov six persons could live in the hospital in 1539,[60] but at Kalundborg in 1564 accommodation was provided for only four inmates of the hospital.[61] In Roskilde, the statutes of the *Duebrødre* hospital of 1478 stipulated that it should have four poor residents and a few school pupils; the abolition of the chantries made it possible to take in two more inmates. In 1569, when the hospital was united with the Holy Spirit and leper hospitals the number of inmates was increased to sixteen.[62] At Mariager the Rosenkrantz family had founded several chantries, which ceased to exist at the Reformation. In 1564 their estates were transferred to the hospital of Horsens, where five persons were to be maintained from part of the revenues; the Rosenkrantzes were to choose the persons in question.[63]

The most ambitious project for an institution which was limited to the sick (and in that sense an infirmary proper) was Claus Denne's St Anne's hospital. The founder had suffered three years' imprisonment (for what reason we do not know) and had made a vow to build a chapel with a house for visitors in honour of God and St Anne. His ideas were supported by Queen Elizabeth, who in 1516 recommended that her subjects contribute to their realisation.[64] Denne was himself a physician, and his institution appears to have worked for some years, until he fell out of grace with the king, and moved with his patients to Sweden, where he had managed to win the support of King Gustavus Vasa. The king allowed him to collect alms in Sweden, where the hospital owned lands.[65] A St Anne's hospital was additionally opened at Aahus in East Scania by 1525,[66] where the year before Frederik I had given his permission to Denne to reopen his hospital in the capital. It was to be built in stone and have a bath; the aim was to care for fifty patients. Admission to the hospital was free, but the institution was to take possession of the belongings of those dying there. Those who recovered were free to take their belongings with them when they left. Besides the infirmary, a guest house for travelling pilgrims was to be established, where they could have a free meal and stay overnight; those who could pay for their sojourn were asked to do so. The running of the institution was to be financed by alms collected from Denmark and Norway.[67]

Denne used his private fortune to realise his ideas, but the alms collected were far from sufficient, and after some years, at the latest in 1530, the hospital had to close. Its property was united with that of the leper hospital and of the Holy Spirit house, where Copenhagen's hospital was set up.[68]

In order to secure sufficient incomes for the hospitals, rather complex unions were sometimes effected. We have already seen that two or more hospitals in the same town could be merged into one, but in some cases the reorganisation was very complex. In Ribe, the former Dominican monastery was transformed in 1543 into a general hospital for the sick and poor. To it were added Ribe's Holy Spirit House, and Ribe's and Kolding's leper hospitals as well as lands in the countryside, probably belonging to a former chantry.[69] More radical was the arrangement made at Aarhus in 1541. The Dominican monastery was to be a general hospital for the sick and poor; to it the property of the Holy Spirit hospitals at Horsens and Randers was transferred, a necessary measure as a mendicant institution normally owned very little land besides the plot upon which it stood. The inmates from Randers and Horsens were to be moved to Aarhus;[70] in this way the relief of their poverty would mean their total isolation from the world in which they once lived.

In this respect the reform was a failure in Jutland; in 1558 the government realised this, asking the bishops and governor of each diocese to examine the conditions of each institution. Where the revenues were insufficient or where it appeared reasonable to reopen the closed hospitals, the possibilities of financing their activities were to be considered.[71] As a consequence of this investigation, hospitals were created at Randers and Kolding, and the hospital at Horsens was reopened; land and revenue formerly belonging to those of Randers and Horsens and transferred to Aarhus Hospital, were given back.[72]

The church statutes of 1542 had introduced a new source of financing, which was used only from the late 1550s: in many cases overseers of hospitals were only appointed if they promised to let the institution inherit their belongings when they died; in return they could live for free in the hospital when they stopped working.[73] One of the earliest appointments was that of Knud Andersen as overseer of the Holy Spirit house and the leper hospital, both at Slagelse, in 1557.[74] The incumbent was at the same time rector of two parish churches, which he was allowed to keep on condition of paying a vicar.[75] Thus, in spite of all good intentions, the Protestant government lapsed back into the late medieval practice of granting part of ecclesiastical revenues to non-residents.[76] A recurring clause in the urban statutes of the Sound region reveal abuse of the Holy Spirit houses, considered as institutions for the poor: the inmates were prohibited from trading unless they paid taxes to the town.[77]

However, the problem was to procure sufficient incomes for the new hospitals, since these new institutions, which were mainly urban, had less real estate than important rural abbeys like Cara Insula or Æbelholt had. When they were closed as religious institutions their landed property was taken over by the Crown or eventually sold to members of the aristocracy. Begging on behalf of hospitals was again allowed, because of shortage of funds, and at the same time the government distinguished clearly between deserving and non-deserving sick. For solely moral reasons, former prostitutes suffering from venereal diseases were not to be admitted into hospital, in order not to encourage others – sin was not to be seen to pay.[78]

PHYSICIANS AND APOTHECARIES

In a few cases like Malmø, Ribe or Slagelse[79] a physician or a surgeon was attached to the new hospitals established after the Reformation, but the government was aware of the general need for competent physicians or surgeons. Free housing or at least a plot for construction was sometimes provided[80] and in smaller towns a surgeon could obtain the right of precedence to patients to be treated.[81] This shows us that although most towns had at least one resident surgeon, it could be difficult for smaller towns to find one.

The government was concerned to attract fully educated physicians; both at Ribe and at Viborg certain revenues were in 1545 reserved for a doctor or *licentiatus* of medicine;[82] in 1563 a certain Peder Sørensen was appointed to Viborg, but before taking up residence he had to study for three years abroad, for example in Italy or France.[83]

The physicians in royal service were obviously the most privileged group: free housing, a decent salary, and sometimes even a salary for teaching in the university;[84] when the eye specialist Jonas Möller wanted to establish himself in Denmark, he was allowed to live in Copenhagen, was given exemption from taxes and other charges and was authorised to work over all Denmark.[85]

The government showed the same concern for apothecaries as for physicians. In 1514 Hans Apoteker at Copenhagen was granted the monopoly of selling claret and ground spices and was exempted from taxes as well.[86] His venture apparently met with limited success, as in 1536 a house in Copenhagen was given to Johan Dich, who obliged himself to open a dispensary by Whitsun 1537.[87] Dich's enterprise seems to have thrived, as ten years later a new apothecary in Copenhagen was recognised; he was given tax exemption and had to rent his predecessor's house; in 1550 he obtained the monopoly of making medicaments.[88] The dispensary's standard declined, and in 1569 two physicians were ordered by the government to undertake a serious inspection, controlling the prices and the quality of the drugs.[89]

Outside the capital it proved more difficult to attract apothecaries. The government recognised the need in 1549, when it authorised Dr Cornelius Hamsfort, physician to the king, to open a dispensary. Dr Hamsfort already had at his disposal a house at Odense belonging to the crown, and he and his descendants were granted exclusive rights to the production of medicaments. If no suitable apothecary could to be found within the family, it was obliged to engage one to run the dispensary. The head of the household using the house was moreover given exemption from town taxes.[90] Hamsfort was eventually succeeded by his son of the same name, who died in 1627.[91]

For as long as the monastery of Cara Insula had existed, it had cared for the sick. In 1556 an apothecary was appointed; he was to have free board, clothes and lodging in the monastery, to which he was to offer his services.[92] This measure reveals that the government recognised the value of the medical tradition of Cara Insula. We can only guess whether or not the government intended to maintain the monastery as a hospital. At all events, after Christian III's death his successor wanted to live part of the year in this excellent region for hunting; so Cara Insula was in 1560 closed, and the bricks were used for the construction of Skanderborg Castle.

HYGIENIC MEASURES

Medieval urban legislation contained several clauses limiting rather than preventing pollution,[93] and sixteenth-century central government was also aware of this problem. In May 1548 the city of Ribe received St Peter's Church and churchyard outside Ribe, since during epidemics burials were only allowed out of town.[94] Six years later, the prior of St Canute's in Odense was ordered to enlarge the building of the school. Like that of Nyborg it was too small in view of the number of pupils, who could not be allowed to sit too close to each other in case of epidemics or other diseases.[95] In April 1562 the central government noticed that many pigs and cows had died in Zealand during the winter, above all because the dead animals were not carried away and buried, thus infecting the sound animals. In order to prevent epidemics in the hotter climate of summer, it was ordered that dead animals had to be removed from any settlement – town or village – immediately and be buried at such a depth that contamination was no longer possible.[96]

Finally, we should not forget also that public authorities took an interest in medicine in other respects. When Henrik Smith of Malmø had a medical treatise translated into Danish, he was granted exclusive rights to print and distribute it for five years,[97] and town courts watched quacks very carefully, as we learn from cases from Malmø in 1553[98] and from Elsinore in 1562.[99] In the Malmø case most cures had succeeded and no further action was taken. At Elsinore the cures had proven ineffectual, so the quack and her husband were on 14 October 1562 ordered to leave Elsinore by Easter 1563.[100]

CONCLUSION

In the distinction between able-bodied and deserving poor, Protestant social policy continued that of the later Middle Ages, and like its medieval counterpart, had to rely heavily on private alms. This circumstance had not been foreseen by the Reformers, but was a consequence of the fact that the richest charitable institutions – the rural monasteries – were not left as charitable endowments but were taken over by the crown or by the aristocracy. A similar situation developed in Scotland, where the Reformers failed to appropriate the patrimony of the old church.[101] In Denmark, only mendicant houses were given to poor relief, but as the Franciscans had been reformed shortly before the Reformation, their real estate consisted mainly of the buildings. Thus, as no poor rates were introduced, the resources available for charity may have diminished; for unknown reasons poor rates were introduced only about 1630, and then only for a few towns.[102] At the same time, if the quantity of available work remained stable, underemployment increased as Catholic holidays were abolished. Moreover, the armies of the sixteenth century consisted mainly of mercenaries who were often disbanded far from home and thus had to beg their way until they found a new war in which to enrol.

Thus the resources available for charity may have diminished as a consequence of the Reformation and of the agreement between aristocracy and crown in appropriating most property formerly belonging to the church; at the same time the need for assistance increased. The manifest concern of Protestant Denmark to use its charitable institutions more efficiently could only remedy the social problem to a very limited extent, and the primary motive for private charity[103] – the urge to save one's soul and to limit its stay in purgatory – had been removed by the change of religion. The circumstance that for the first fifty years following the Reformation public charities prevailed, whereas after 1586 their leading position was taken over by private endowments,[104] shows clearly that public relief had been inadequate and that private donors began to realise this half a century after the Reformation.

NOTES

1 For a summary of Poul Helgesen's ideas on poor relief, see Thomas Riis, 'L'assistance aux pauvres et la Réforme danoise', *Dacia*, 52, 1986, 13. The text itself, 'Huore krancke, mijslige, saare, arme og fattige menneskir schule tracteris oc besorges: een kort vnderwijsning aff Broder Paulo Helie', was published in Marius Kristensen (ed.) *Skrifter af Paulus Helie*, vol. 3, Copenhagen 1933, 3–37; it was first printed in Copenhagen in 1528.

2 Thomas Riis, 'Religion and Early Modern Social Welfare', in Emily Albu Hanawalt and Carter Lindberg (eds) *Through the Eye of a Needle. Judeo-Christian roots of social welfare*, Kirksville, Missouri 1994, 194–5. Moreover, St Paul had written that whoever does not work shall not eat (*II Thess.* 3, 10).

3 Eino Jutikkala, 'Labour policy and urban proletariat in Sweden-Finland', in Thomas Riis (ed.) *Aspects of Poverty in Early Modern Europe II*, Odense 1986, 135–6; Bronislaw Geremek, *La Potence ou la Pitié. L'Europe et les pauvres du Moyen Age à nos jours*, Paris 1987, 96, 110–1.

4 *Den Danske Rigslovgivning indtil 1400*, ed. Erik Kroman, Copenhagen 1971, 231–2, c. 1/7/1354 no. 3.

5 E.g. the firepan granted to the Malmø Franciscans; the town government made a plot available for the storage of coal for it, cf. *Malmø Stadsbog 1503–1548*, ed. E. Kroman, Copenhagen 1995, 4 (16/11/1503).

6 Cf. e.g. Jean-Pierre Gutton, 'Les pauvres face à leur pauvreté: le cas français 1500–1800', in Thomas Riis (ed.) *Aspects of Poverty in Early Modern Europe II*, Odense 1986, 95–6.

7 Urban statute 6/1/1522 art. 88 and 92, rural statute c. 6/1/1522 art. 120 (*Den danske Rigslovgivning 1513–23*, ed. A. Andersen, Copenhagen, 1991, 78–80, 129–30, 195, 243).

8 Urban statute art. 91, rural statute art. 116 (*Den danske Rigslovgivning 1513–23*, 79, 130, 194, 243).

9 Urban statute art. 93, rural statute art. 112 (*Den danske Rigslovgivning 1513–23*, 80, 130–1, 192–3, 244). The rural statute exempted from the right to beg homicides collecting money for their fines (art. 113) and those who had wilfully set fire to their own house (art. 114) (*Den danske Rigslovgivning 1513–23*, 193, 242–3).

10 See Chapter 7 of this volume.

11 Franz Irsigler, 'Bettler und Dirnen in der städtischen Gesellschaft des 14.–16. Jahrhunderts', in Thomas Riis (ed.) *Aspects of Poverty in Early Modern Europe II*, 182–4.

12 Cf. Charles Wilson, 'The other Face of Mercantilism', *Transactions of the Royal Historical Society* 5th series, IX, 1959, *passim*.

13 J. L. A. Kolderup-Rosenvinge (ed.) *Samling af gamle danske Love*, IV, Copenhagen 1824, 166.

14 See e.g. *Kancelliets Brevbøger vedrørende Danmarks indre Forhold*, ed. C. F. Bricka *et al.*, Copenhagen 1885, ff. 8/1/1552 (two letters).

15 *Kancelliets. Brevbøger* 2/1/1557; Secher, *Corpus Constitutionum Daniæ*, II, 582–3, 17/12/1590.

16 Secher, *Corpus Constitutionum Daniæ* II, *loc. cit.*
17 *ibid.*, I, Copenhagen 1887–8, 172–4, (18/11/1561), 457–8 (6/9/ 1570) and II, 532–6 (31/5/1589).
18 *ibid.*, I, 42–4.
19 *ibid.*, I, 536–7, 540–1 (19/5 and 28/5/1573), 591–3 (14/7/1574); *ibid.*, II, 4–5 for Copenhagen (28/2/1576), 338–9 (7/9/1583 for the *len* of Haderslev.
20 *ibid.*, II, 20–1 (13/8/1576).
21 *Danske Kirkelove*, ed. Holger Fr. Rørdam, II, Copenhagen 1886, 353–4 (19/6/1582).
22 Secher, *Corpus Constitutionum Daniæ*, II, 497–508. Christian II's urban and rural statutes, if introduced, had been abolished soon after his fall in 1523.
23 *Diplomaticum Danicum*, I, 3, ed. C.A. Christensen, Copenhagen, 1976–7, no. 52.
24 Marianne Johansen in *Køge Bys Historie*, I, Køge 1985, 54–5.
25 Troels Dahlerup, 'Den sociale forsorg og reformationen i Danmark', *Historie. Jyske Samlinger*, Ny rk. XIII, 1979–81, 200; Kr. Erslev, *Danmarks Len og Lensmænd i det Sextende Aarhundrede (1513–96)*, Copenhagen 1879, 24, 148–51; for the secularisation of the rural monasteries, see 144–63.
26 See the list of dissolved Franciscan convents and their later uses in Thomas Riis, 'L'assistance aux pauvres et la Réforme danoise', *Dacia*, LII, 1986, 11–12.
27 Dahlerup, *op. cit.*, 203–6.
28 E.g. *Diplomaticum Danicum*, IV, 3, ed. Thomas Riis, Copenhagen 1993, nos 92 and 96–7 (22/9/1386 and earlier).
29 See, for example, the foundation of an altar in the Cathedral of Ribe, *ibid.*, no. 371 (3/4/1388).
30 Kr. Isager, *Skeletfundene ved Øm Kloster*, Copenhagen 1936 (Cara Insula); Vilh. Møller-Christensen, *Bogen om Æbelholt Kloster*, Copenhagen 1958.
31 The last nun died as late as in the 1620s in the convent of Maribo.
32 *Danmarks Kirker*, II: Frederiksborg Amt 3, Copenhagen 1970, 1416–7; J. P. Trap, *Danmark*, VIII, 2, Copenhagen 1964, 600.
33 *Danske Kirkelove*, ed. Holger Fr. Rørdam I, Copenhagen 1883, 203–4 (ecclesiastical statute 4/5/1542 art. 19–20). See also the proposed arrangement at Copenhagen in 1530 (Kr. Erslev and W. Mollerup (eds) *Kong Frederik den Førstes danske Registranter*, Copenhagen 1879, 268–9).
34 Confirmation dated 23/6/1514, in P. F. Suhm (ed.) *Nye Samlinger til den Danske Historie,*, I, Copenhagen 1792, 66.
35 *Regesta Diplomatica Historiae Danicae*, 1st series I–II; 2nd series I–II, Copenhagen 1847–1907 (henceforth *Reg. Dan.*), nos. 5545 (21/2 1513) and *9875 (22/2/1513)).
36 P. F. Suhm *et al.* (eds) *Samlinger til den Danske Historie*, II, 1, Copenhagen 1784, 157–8 (3/8/1517), 160–2 (8/12/1517); Reg. Dan. no. *10,244 (12/12/1517). Kr. Erslev and W. Mollerup (eds) *Danske Kancelliregistranter 1535–50*, Copenhagen 1881–2, 75–6,

(10/12/1538). Lepers were mentioned at Aalborg still in 1552, *Kancelliets Brevbøger*, 28/5/1552.

37 *Kong Frederik den Førstes danske Registranter*, 3–4 (Ribe, 13/5/1523), 8–9 (Copenhagen 17/6/1523) and 14 (Næstved 1/8/1523).

38 *ibid.*, 257 (12/7/1530). *Danske Kancelliregistranter 1535–50*, 160 (undated, probably April-May 1541).

39 Hans de Hofman (ed.) *Samlinger af Publique og Private Stiftelser, Fundationer og Gavebreve...*, II, Copenhagen 1756, 103–5 (royal letters of 1515 and 1541).

40 Aage Andersen (ed.) *Den danske Rigslovgivning 1513–23*, Copenhagen 1991, 79–80, 130 (town statute, 6/1/1522, art. 91).

41 *ibid.*, 194, 243 (rural statute art. 116).

42 J. Lindbæk and G. Stemann, *De danske Helligaandsklostre. Fremstilling og Aktstykker*, Copenhagen 1906, 4–17.

43 Alfr. Krarup and Johs. Lindbæk (eds) *Acta Pontificum Danica* V, Copenhagen 1913, no. 3339 (21/2/1493).

44 *Kong Frederik den Førstes danske Registranter*, 181 (8/10/1528).

45 *ibid.*, 255 (4/7/1530).

46 *ibid.*, 207–8 (5/6/1529).

47 This applied above all to the monasteries of the Franciscans; see Thomas Riis, 'L'assistance aux pauvres et la Réforme danoise', *Dacia*, LII, 1986, 11–12.

48 *Kancelliets Brevbøger*, 29/9/1555 cf. 12/7/1556.

49 *Danske Magazin*, 4th series, IV, Copenhagen 1878, 147–8.

50 *Danske Magazin*, 4th series, I, Copenhagen 1864, 327 (28/9/1547). See also the fate of the Scottish endowments at Copenhagen and Elsinore, Thomas Riis, *Should Auld Acquaintance Be Forgot... Scottish–Danish Relations c. 1450–1707*, Odense 1989, I, 196, 240–1.

51 Suhms, *Nye Samlinger*, I, 166.

52 *Kong Frederik den Førstes danske Registranter*, 440, 461.

53 *Kancelliets Brevbøger*, 29/7/1570 (confirmation).

54 *ibid.*, 4/6/1552 and *ibid.*, 23/2/1557.

55 *ibid.*, 12/7/1561.

56 *ibid.*, 12/1/1562.

57 *ibid.*, 4/4/1563.

58 Suhms *Samlinger*, II 1, 147 (10/7/1516).

59 *Kong Frederik den Førstes danske Registranter*, 434–5, perhaps from July 1532.

60 *Danske Kancelliregistranter 1535–1550*, 90–1 (16/6/1539).

61 *Kancelliets Brevbøger*, 29/4/1564.

62 *Danmarks Kirker*, III: Københavns Amt 1, Copenhagen 1944, 161; *Danske Kancelliregistranter 1535–50*, 257 (27/12/1542); *Kancelliets Brevbøger*, 30/8/1569; Rørdam (ed.) *Danske Kirkelove*, II, 145 f. (24/8/1570).

63 *Kancelliets Brevbøger*, 19/3/1564.

64 *Reg. Dan.*, no. *10,125 (11/3/1516).

65 *Reg. Dan.*, no. *11,001 (11/9/1523). On Claus Denne in general, see Erik Arup, *Danmarks Historie*, II, Copenhagen 1932, 309–10 and

Bjørn Kornerup in *Dansk Biografisk Leksikon*, III, Copenhagen 1979, 614.

66 *Kong Frederik den Førstes danske Registranter*, 75 (17/8/1525), confirmation of statutes.

67 *ibid.*, 57–9 (25/9/1524).

68 *ibid.*, 268–9 (August 1530).

69 *Danske Kancelliregistranter 1535–1550*, 267–8 (12/10/1543); *Danmarks Kirker*, XIX: Ribe Amt 2, Copenhagen 1984, 819.

70 *Danske Kancelliregistranter 1535–1550*, 206–7; *Danske Magazin*, 3rd series VI, 312.

71 *Kanc. Brevbøger*, 3/10/1558.

72 *ibid.*, 6/12, 10/12 and 12/12 1558 (Randers), 15/12/1558 (Kolding), 8/5/1560 (Horsens).

73 Church statutes of 1542 art. 18 (Rørdam (ed.) *Danske Kirkelove*, I, 203).

74 *Kanc. Brevbøger*, 19/10/1557.

75 *ibid.*, 23/5/1558.

76 A similar arrangement was made in 1558 when the bishop of Viborg obtained part of the rector's incomes of Vinkel and Ring parishes (*ibid.*, 6/12/1558).

77 *Danmarks Gamle Købstadlovgivning*, ed. Erik Kroman, III, Copenhagen 1955, 89: Copenhagen 1443 V art. 41; *ibid.*, 144: Elsinore early 16th c. art. 69; *ibid.*, IV, Copenhagen 1961, 87 Malmø 1487 art. 52, 138 Landskrona art. 51, 285 Halmstad 1498 art. 57.

78 *Danske Magazin*, 4th series I, 194 (27/3/1546).

79 *Malmø (Stadsbok) 1503–48*, ed. Erik Kroman, Copenhagen 1965, 145–6 (11/12/1538); Ribe: *Danske Kancelliregistranter 1535–1550*, 37 (16/3/1537); Slagelse: *ibid.*, 160 (April-May 1541).

80 *Danske Kancelliregistranter 1535–1550*, 37 (Ribe 1537), 160 (Slagelse 1541), 220 (Ribe 1542); *Kancelliets Brevbøger*, 5/1/1555 and 21/12/1555 Ribe, cf. *ibid.*, 30/9/1559.

81 *Danske Kancelliregistranter 1535–1550*, 334 (30/8/1547, Landskrona); *Danske Magazin*, 4th series V, Copenhagen 1884, 326 (23/9/1550, Ystad); *ibid.*, 4th series VI, Copenhagen 1886, 156–7 (5/10/1550 Aarhus).

82 *Danske Kancelliregistranter 1535–1550*, 274–6 (19/1 and 20/2/1545). At the same time a physician/apothecary settled at Schleswig, but was dismissed in 1546, cf. Vilh. Møller-Christensen and Albert Gjedde, 'Det medicinske Fakultet 1479–1842', in *Københavns Universitet 1479–1979, VII: det lægevidenskabelige Fakultet*, Copenhagen 1979, 15. On surgeons' crafts, see *ibid.*, 1–3.

83 *Kancelliets Brevbøger*, 28/10/1563.

84 See e.g. the letters of appointment for Dr Peder Capiteyn 3/1/1547 (*Danske Kancelliregistranter 1535–50*, 325–6), for Dr Jacob Bording 25/5/1557 (*Kanc. Brevbøger*), for Dr Cornelius Hamsfort 13/6/1551 and 26/2/1554 (*ibid.*) and for the surgeon Robert Geyspusch, who like Hamsfort did not teach in the university, 27/4/1556 (*ibid.*).

85 *Kancelliets Brevbøger*, 23/2/1570.

86 Suhm, *Nye Samlinger*, II 1, 116 (4/3/1514).

87 *Danske Kancelliregistranter 1535–50*, 34 (11/12/1536).
88 *ibid.*, for Villum Unno 303 and 441 (15/9/1546 and 25/3/1550).
89 *Kancelliets Brevbøger*, 5/3/1569. See also R. Kruse, *Lægemiddelpriserne i Danmark Indtil 1645*Copenhagen 1991, 59–64.
90 *Danske Kancelliregistranter 1535–50*, 414 (24/4/1549).
91 R. Paulli, in *Dansk Biografisk Leksikon*, V, Copenhagen 1980, 535–6.
92 *Kanc. Brevbøger*, 5/7/1556.
93 Cf. Thomas Riis, 'Istituzioni e crescita urbana in Europa: problemi di metodo', *Storia della Città*, 43, 1988, 43.
94 *Danske Magazin*, 4th series II, 81.
95 *Kanc. Brevbøger*, 4/12/1554.
96 *ibid.*, 28/4/1562 (three letters). In Copenhagen dead animals had to be removed only once a week (*ibid.*). Similar measures: inhabitants of plague stricken towns were prohibited from travelling (V.A. Secher (ed.) *Corpus Constitutionum Daniae*, II, Copenhagen 1889–90 117–8, 152, 26/9 1578, 27/12/1579). Entry into houses of victims of plague and selling of old clothes forbidden during the time of plague (*ibid.*, 618–9, 11/8/1592).
97 *Kanc. Brevbøger*, 18/5/1555.
98 Einar Bager (ed.) *Malmø Stadsbog 1549–59*, Copenhagen 1972, 132–3.
99 Karen Hjorth and Erik Kroman (eds) *Helsingør Stadsbog 1554–55, 1559–60 og 1561–65*, Copenhagen 1981, 191–2.
100 Intervention against quacks could also be undertaken in order to protect the interests of surgeons, cf. V. A. Secher (ed.) *Corpus Constitutionum Daniae*, II, 124–5, no. 146 (10/1/1579).
101 T. C. Smout, *A History of the Scottish People 1560–1830*, Glasgow 1972, 85.
102 See Chapter 7 of this volume.
103 It is further a question of whether Denmark's economy was so advanced as to allow a greater number of charitable endowments like those known abroad; cf. W. K. Jordan, *Philanthropy in England 1480–1660*, London 1959, 368, table 1. Jordan's figures of charitable endowments 1480–1540 show that 15 per cent were for poor relief and social rehabilitation. The overwhelming majority of Danish endowments took the form of chantries which after the Reformation were suppressed or modified, only sometimes for charitable purposes.
104 See Chapter 7, table 1, of this volume.

The wrath of God

Christian IV and poor relief in the wake of the Danish intervention in the Thirty Years' War

E. Ladewig Petersen

On 1 May 1630 the magistracy in Copenhagen took over a former clerical meeting house in Silkegade which Christian IV had donated to the city as a centre for its newly re-organised poor relief. The inscription placed over the entrance to the building proclaimed that this was 'a charitable house for the poor, a holy house, which King Christian IV had instituted for the proper care of the poor in Copenhagen'.[1] This re-organisation of public charity in the capital during 1629–30 was followed by new arrangements for poor relief in at least three of the country's major towns, Ribe, Odense and Viborg, while no similar arrangements appear to have been made for the countryside.

The inscription ended with the king's motto, *regnas firmat pietas* – 'piety strengthens the kingdoms' (Denmark and Norway). Even if the king's motto quickly became the target for popular wit, for the king – God's annointed shepherd of his flock – it was meant in earnest, not least after his rash and disastrous intervention in the Thirty Years' War which had damaged not only his personal standing, but also his realm and the evangelical cause. It is evident that Christian IV, from around 1629, convinced of his own pure faith and Christ's redeeming grace, deliberately set about having himself portrayed in both texts and pictures as a parallel to Christ, betrayed by Judas and convicted and humiliated by Pilate and the Pharisees.[2] Contemplation caused him to expiate and atone, but not to question the rightfulness and justice of his royal-evangelical mission.

Strangely enough Christian IV, unlike Gustavus Adolphus of Sweden, had never prepared his subjects for his evangelical crusade in Germany through similar, massive anti-Catholic propaganda. Instead, he had limited his attempts to mould public opinion to general days of prayer, and not until he issued a statute against 'cursing and swearing' in 1623 did he warn the general public that such blasphemous behaviour inevitably invoked 'the certain signs of God's wrath', such as dearth, war, rebellion and plague, as could already be observed in neighbouring countries. The defeat in 1626 and the subsequent occupation of Jutland by Imperial Catholic troops served to actualise these and even worse apocalyptic visions for the Danish population. A poignant feeling pervaded, of having offended God, and that His anger and punishment might only be averted though penance and prayer.[3] This sense of sin and atonement imbued not only the government's legislation but also the general attitude of the population in the years leading up to 1630. It probably found its strongest expression in the important statute of 1629 about 'the office and authority of the church over unrepentant sinners'.[4] The idea that God's judgement and punishment was imminent played a prominent part, even if the statute was primarily concerned with the practical implementation of church discipline, penance, prayer and confession, including the threat of severe sanctions from ecclesiastical as well as lay authorities against those who did not conform. The statute, with its ferocious Old Testament-inspired language, closely corresponded to the disciplinary reform programme implemented within the post-Tridentine Catholic Church, with its call for pious penitence, punishment and repentance under the supervision of the proper authorities.[5]

It was, however, not only the losing side which was affected by these apocalyptic expectations, having been afflicted by 'God's just punishment'. This pervading sentiment of gloom and doom while the Day of Judgement was seen to be rapidly approaching dominated the Catholic powers as well. *Dies irae, dies illa*, the day of wrath, when God would reduce the world to dust and ashes because of its sins and lack of piety, was also central to the Catholic mentality of the age. Evidently the Catholic powers, the Emperor, the League, the Curia and Spain could interpret the defeat of the Protestants as proof of the justice of their cause, but with victory came the obligation to return the apostate heretics to the Catholic fold. These concerns resulted initially in the infamous Edict of Restitution of 1629, which intended to regain much of what had been lost to the Protestants since the Religious Peace of Augsburg in 1555, not only in terms of ecclesiastical property but also in terms of souls.[6] 'The crown belongs to him who fights for justice' was of course the motto of Emperor Ferdinand II.

The confessional confrontation probably reached its peak around 1630. The experience of war, dearth, plague and accelerating social tensions was far from restricted to Denmark,[7] but became a common experience in most of Northern and Western Europe at a time when the growing conflict on the continent made ever greater demands on human as well as material resources. Dearth, plague and a crisis in popular religion and perception created serious problems for lay and ecclesiastical authorities across Europe while a need for increased control and greater order came to be seen to be imperative.

A proposal from 1627 for the reform and centralisation of all hospitals in Denmark demonstrates that Christian IV, like most of his contemporaries, distinguished between the resident, deserving poor and the vagrant undeserving poor. In stern and simplistic terms the king pointed out that those inmates in hospitals who could hear and perceive and those 'who had never learnt anything when they were children' (i.e. piety and regular work), and similar 'godless inmates', should be expelled immediately, even if they were invalids; vagrants were to be imprisoned and forced to work. The only deserving inmates of the hospitals were those who were 'demented and mad' and 'the deaf'.[8] Strangely enough, the king, in this intemperate outburst against the undeserving poor, appears to have forgotten most of those traditionally considered deserving in this period, such as the old and infirm, orphans and invalids.

The distinction between the deserving and undeserving poor had its roots in the canon law of the later Middle Ages, which had dealt in detail with the issue of how far the biblical obligation towards the poor should be taken, and the dangers of forfeiting the souls of local people, as well as strangers. The result had been the distinction on the one hand between the local, deserving poor who were demonstrably unable to look after themselves, let alone work, and on the other, sturdy vagrants who avoided their Christian obligation to work and provide for themselves, something which the late medieval church attached great importance to.[9] Even if governments added new aspects and elements to the way they dealt with poverty and poor relief, especially in the form of control and punishment, it is an open question to what extent these changes introduced during the sixteenth- and seventeenth centuries significantly changed the way the poor and their relief was considered and handled by early modern authorities. New impulses in this field appear to have been closely linked to the growing confessional conflicts and the accelerating social and economic hardship, which served to make the salvation of souls an imperative while the preservation of law and order became a necessity.

The prospect of 'full employment' had, at least, remained a possibility in the plague-ravaged Europe of the fourteenth century, as long as the deserving poor were cared for;[10] the population increase of the sixteenth century, however, made a mockery of this dream. The means of production of the period were simply unable to absorb the population surplus, which by itself generated a rapidly expanding group of social outcasts who were forced into vagrancy and chronic unemployment, in a wretched existence at the margins of society. Another equally important explanation may be found in the distorted age distribution within the population of early modern Europe, with children comprising 35–40 per cent of the total population, and less than half the population being within the labour-active age group from fifteen to sixty years, as a result of high mortality and recurring epidemics.[11] It is hardly surprising then, that the myriad of poor and vagrants we are confronted with in this period are generally portrayed as children, single women, cripples, the worn-out elderly, and, of course, vagabonds, charlatans, not to mention – a sign of the times – the depraved and crippled soldiers.

In a period which was characterised by a growing social polarisation between rich and poor and which witnessed an increase in criminality and lawlessness, the deep concern of most post-Reformation legislation to try to separate the corn from the chaff should not surprise us. It was of paramount importance for the authorities to try to limit unavoidable local poverty while simultaneously trying to prevent and eventually criminalise vagrancy. In this context it was a natural progression that begging came to be associated by the governing classes in Protestant Europe with violence, theft and lawlessness. Such groups were perceived to be anti-social, often sustaining a separate subculture and identity detached from the rest of society. These negative views were regularly reinforced through the recurrent outbreaks of famine – especially in the years around 1630 – which in each case necessitated government intervention to prevent disturbances and food riots among the poor of the region, who more often than not were supported by the growing number of vagrants.

In Northern, Protestant Europe the new social legislation was characterised by a mixture of local welfare provisions supplemented by increasingly coercive measures directed against vagrants in particular, while in Italy and Spain post-Tridentine Catholicism encouraged the creation of new and more dynamic charitable societies. England, where the wealth and possessions of the Catholic Church were confiscated by the Crown in connection with the Reformation, with little or no consideration for the loss of relief to the poor, pioneered the introduction of a compulsory tax, the poor rate, raised on a parochial basis from 1572 onwards, and the introduction of workhouses and houses of correction, starting with Bridewell in London in 1552 and later followed by similar institutions in many provincial towns, which were intended to be 'houses of production' where the deviant poor could be taught a trade while producing goods; furthermore towards the end of the sixteenth century the poor benefited by a considerable increase in private charity and donations.[12] It is noteworthy that the English example of establishing houses of correction was initially only taken up in the United Provinces, and then not until the 1590s, from where it then spread to the Baltic and Germany.

Developments in Denmark followed the general European pattern closely. As opposed to England the government in Denmark made sure that local hospitals were continued in the wake of the Reformation. Income belonging to such institutions was retained and in many cases supplemented by the crown. In the towns it was administered by the newly appointed local hospital supervisors, while funds for the poor were controlled by the local minister in collaboration with local government.[13] From 1537 the division between the deserving poor, whom society was obliged to support, and the undeserving, able-bodied poor, whose claim to assistance should be rejected, was legally established in Denmark; this division was further enhanced in 1558 when it became possible to employ such able-bodied beggars and poor in forced labour. These trends were further cemented through the comprehensive poor law of 1587 which legally enforced the practice of forced labour, and which requested registration of the poor locally, in order that the deserving poor could be supplied with badges authorising their begging. This was done in order to supplement the often inadequate resources regularly collected for the poor in the parish churches or on special occasions.

Thus we know that the government began using forced labour at the Bremerholm naval dockyard before 1570. Not only criminals were conscripted for this purpose, but also able-bodied vagrants who were found begging. Royal administrators were regularly ordered to arrest such people; during 1646 around 154 forced labourers were employed at Bremerholm, receiving only small sums to cover expenses for food and basic necessities.[14] This practice of forcing the able-bodied poor to work was greatly expanded in the first years of the reign of Christian IV when vagabonds were regularly condemned to forced labour on the king's many and extensive building works on the fortifications along the border with Sweden. This policy found its strongest institutional expression in the creation of the house of correction, *Tugthuset* in Copenhagen in 1605.

This institution, together with the 'Childrens' House for Poor Orphans', which was founded in 1619, combined the idea of using the poor and marginalised as forced labour while simultaneously trying to re-socialise them through education and training, not least by giving talented and willing poor children the chance to learn a craft; 'for His Royal Majesty's profit' – a conscious economic policy was thus intertwined with an 'employment policy' shaped by mercantilism.[15] These institutions, which regularly housed between 300 and 500 convicted criminals and children, were, of course, typical of the age even if they never succeeded in achieving the government's objectives. In spite of costing the government at least 8,000 thalers annually in the years from 1630 to 1646, the orphanage and the house of correction always retained the interest and favour of Christian IV.

The statute of 1587 had already used an impressive array of abusive language against vagrants in particular and the undeserving poor in general. Terms such as theft by 'healthy and able-bodied beggars', who steal 'the alms of God from other, deserving poor', and who blaspheme against God by refusing to work, were repeatedly used, pointing out the dangers to society of beggars, supplicants, hags, cast-off or sham soldiers, scoundrels, charlatans, and godless and blaspheming packs of thieves, among others, who acted with 'roguishness and combined obstruction with theft and ungodly actions' such as 'swindling, witchcraft, deception, and fraudulency' in order to compel people under the threat of violence to give them alms. However, no detailed evidence for the existence of a 'proletarian subculture' exists, but even so the reaction of the magistracy in the town of Aarhus to the 1587 statute was probably typical, when it used the opportunity to banish no less than 128 beggars – thieves, charlatans and whores – of whom eighty-three were women, forty-one men and four children.[16]

That such attitudes to the non-resident poor could be combined as a matter of course with a spectacular stinginess in the employment of a paid and salaried workforce, constitutes a paradox not only in Danish history of this period but also in European history. It was, of course, implicit in the way feudal society was structured that the villeinage of the peasantry was free of charge, but preserved accounts from private and entailed estates clearly show that copyholders were obliged to take on all casual and unskilled work, while salaried work was limited to a minimum of skilled craftsmen who were indispensable. Undoubtedly the need and wish to keep expenses down promoted such policies among the gentry, even if they were irreconcilable with the duties prescribed by the legislation. However, this dilemma, if realised by peasants and copyholders, never found public expression.

To the extent that salaried work mattered, Denmark did not experience the same fall in real wages as did other parts of Europe in this period as a consequence of the expansion of the labour force and the subsequent unemployment, but it is noteworthy that the Danish government in the period 1606–55 (and later) laid down scales for maximum wages and emphasised the obligation of vagrants to work. The terms of reference remained severe, but just as remarkably and inexplicably the scales for maximum wages were increasing – normally an indication of labour shortages. This is especially strange when it is borne in mind that such statutes generally sought to ensure that the lowest possible wages were offered in order to encourage the idle to work hard simply in order to survive.[17]

In terms of social history it is of interest to note that many rural people preferred irregular work and begging to long-term employment as servants; consequently, the statute of 1619 lumped servants who opted for idleness and begging with vagrants: both groups were to be punished through forced labour. Thus it is evident from the statutes that the boundaries between the poorer sections of the rural population and vagrant beggars and criminals were fluid. They also show us that by the beginning of the seventeenth century it was no longer possible to absorb the population surplus by establishing new copyholds – as had been done in Jutland and Scania – or by providing houses on the islands with or without smallholdings attached. Christian IV's coercive measures and the creation of the house of correction and orphanage were undoubtedly inspired by developments abroad, as was his suggestion of 1627 to establish a general hospital for the whole realm which would take over all funds hitherto dedicated to local hospitals.[18] The king imagined that such a scheme would make it possible to cater for more than a further hundred deserving inmates. Thus the indications are twofold: first, the government keenly sought a solution to vagrancy and begging, second, and possibly of greater significance, increased poverty was causing acute social and political problems.

Considering the impact and relevance of poverty it is remarkable that the statute of 1629, concerned with ecclesiastical discipline, did not refer to it at all, even if its introduction focused strongly on the nation's sins against God and demanded an iron discipline be imposed on the population. The reason, however, materialised a couple of months later when the Council recommended the king to issue a grave injunction to all local authorities, emphasising their duty to enforce the prescribed initiatives of the 1587 statute against beggars and vagrants. The Council found that the prescriptions laid down in the original statute were adequate and difficult to improve.[19]

In spite of this advice, the following November Christian IV issued a 'good, Christian decree and ordinance for the resident poor and beggars in Copenhagen' in honour of God and for the solace of the poor. Apart from the above-mentioned meeting house for silkweavers, the king donated the sum of 23,150 thalers, consisting of 'altar money, capital and interest', in order 'better to support and further this institution with God's graceful assistance'.[20] The immediate cost of such grand benevolence was, however, not too costly for the king, since most of the money came from old loans and outstanding claims on members of the nobility and burghers. But that the cause was one which received Christian IV's urgent and continuous attention can be seen from the energy and persistence with which he pursued the matter. Thus leading members of the administration felt obliged to support it personally, the Lord Chamberlain Frantz Rantzau and the Chancellor Christen Friis donating 1,000 and 500 thalers respectively.

It is noteworthy that Rantzau and Friis justified their donations by pointing to their residency in Copenhagen, as a consequence of their service to the king. Apparently they considered themselves part of, or associated with, the civic community. The fact that the arrangements they put in place for their donations, namely that the interest should be distributed among the poor on a quarterly basis, anticipated the king's final ordinance, may indicate that their association with this enterprise was close indeed. It can be seen from the instructions Christian IV issued to the committee, consisting of members of the Copenhagen magistracy and clerics, who had been requested to deal with this issue, that they were expected to keep their recommendations within the existing legislation, 'only suggesting what, according to Christian tradition and the time, might be improved'.[21]

The Copenhagen decree of 1630 was in many ways innovative, even if only in parts. The generous sums made available for poor relief in the city – interest from around 60,000 thalers, supplemented with regular voluntary donations and weekly collections in the parish churches for 'the deserving poor' – made it possible to support the poor through quarterly disbursements while simultaneously forbidding begging. Furthermore, the decree placed supervision of the relief of the poor in Copenhagen in the hands of a standing committee, consisting of the bishop, the university's leading professor of theology and two of the city's burghermasters. The direct administration and day-to-day distribution of alms fell to a board of three ministers who were assisted by a small group of salaried officers. They dealt directly with the poor, administered the properties belonging to the charities, helped the able-bodied poor find work (mainly weaving), and sought to exclude vagrants and the undeserving poor from support, often assisted by the 'leaders of the poor' – 'the beggar-kings'.

It is, however, remarkable that the king's initiative was limited to Copenhagen, even if the situation in the capital was in need of urgent attention. That similar setups were introduced in a handful of provincial towns – excluding the countryside – was, as far as we can see, due to local initiatives coming from royal administrators and bishops, who undoubtedly had been inspired by the undertakings in the capital. This was certainly the case for Ribe and Odense where the timing, as well as the content of the re-organisation of poor relief, demonstrate their dependence on developments in Copenhagen. Concerning the other provincial towns, we only know that by 1639 Viborg had a 'voluntary poor relief system', but unfortunately nothing further is known about the exact details.[22]

In Ribe the royal administrator Albert Skeel of Fussingø, and the bishop, Jens Dinesen Jersin, considered the situation insufferable 'with great disorder caused by sturdy beggars'; similar worries affected the royal administrator in Odense, Henning Valkendorf of Glorup and his ecclesiastical colleague the Bishop Hans Mikkelsen.

Nevertheless, the re-organisation of poor relief followed very different avenues in the two towns. Ribe already possessed considerable funds for charitable purposes ('The Guild', hospital donations, capital in the common chest, etc.) which were now supplemented through voluntary contributions, especially from the town's merchants who promised to pay around 1,570 thalers annually. Accordingly it became possible, as in the capital, to register all the needy, including schoolchildren, and to forbid begging.[23]

Since the Reformation, Odense had benefited from possessing a rather well equipped hospital in the former Franciscan monastery; unfortunately the town's magistracy had lost control over the hospital in 1619 and did not regain its administrative power, after prolonged wrangling, until 1635–6. Already during 1630 the magistracy had tried to survey the hospital's existing or new donations, not least after a number of private individuals had donated considerable sums, such as Christen Friis, master of St Knud's monastery, in particular. As early as 1631 Valkendorf informed the king about the considerable popular resistance to and disturbances in Odense directed against the new system of poor relief introduced by the magistracy with the assent of the community. The new system of poor relief in Odense, to which Christian IV gave his assent in 1632, centralised the available funds for relief as had been done in Copenhagen, but as opposed to Ribe the king prescribed an annual poor rate of 800 thalers. But the local resistance continued, especially among craftsmen. Even after fifty-two inhabitants had been pursued through the courts for public disturbances and revolt, it proved impossible for the magistracy to put this decision into practice; the matter was left for the royal administrator, Valkendorf, to deal with. He introduced a new system which was near impossible to distinguish from the original. Thus he retained a poor rate, as originally planned. Everyone was to contribute according to their wealth and income; but the distribution principle followed that already known in other towns.[24]

These reforms were undoubtedly necessary and depended on the initiative of local as well as central government. All their arrangements shared a dependance on voluntary or compulsory payments of regular poor rates. In principle the reforms introduced new methods for making funds available for the poor, but in practice they fell well short of what was needed. No-one questioned the traditional split between the deserving poor and the undeserving, sturdy vagrants or the narrow geographical limitations which were applied. It is, however, significant that the authorities expected, through the centralisation of alms, the introduction of poor rates and a consolidation of the power of the local lay and ecclesiastical authorities, to be able not only to restrain the lawful and licensed local poor, but particularly to exclude the alien and unwanted poor from the towns.

A rough estimate would indicate that the considerable, centralised funds in Copenhagen (excluding the already mentioned clerical meeting house, *Vartov* and several poorhouses) generated an annual income of around 4,000 thalers. It has been estimated that between eleven and nineteen *skilling* was needed to support one poor person per week in this period, at a time when a workman on one of the king's many fortifications would have earned between four and six times as much per week – a considerable difference, even bearing in mind the very different physical conditions the two groups were exposed to. If this estimate is correct, then between 400 and 670 poor, constituting somewhere between 1.6 and 2.7 per cent of 25,000, which by then must have been the population size of the fast-growing capital.[25]

Similarly, the supervisors of poor relief in Odense had a capital of more than 8,300 thalers at their disposal, nearly half of which consisted of various donations from Christen Friis while a slightly smaller amount had been received from the burghers of the town. According to the statute the interest was to be distributed in weekly sums of between eight and twelve *skilling* to 100 poor led by two 'well paid beggar-kings'.[26] Again this would have been enough to support 2–3 per cent of the population. In Ribe however, where the contributions were voluntary, 3–4 per cent could be supported, even if the weekly disbursements were lower.[27] As already mentioned, Viborg had introduced a 'voluntary poor rate' during the 1630s which generated 200 thalers annually. A similar sum appears to have come from collections at the annual meetings of the Jutland nobility (*landsting*) if the sum from 1639 is anything to go by. Thus it would appear that Viborg – a market town of around 3,000 – would have been able to provide a similar percentage of its population with similar weekly sums in poor relief as was the case in Odense. That these figures may have been typical for the alms collected and distributed in most towns is confirmed by the information we have from the small town of Skælskør.[28]

Apart from such outdoor relief, most towns also benefited from the indoor relief provided by hospitals, which in some cases, such as that of Odense, were supposed to cater for the poor of the local diocese. However, it would appear that rural areas only benefited in exceptional cases from such institutions, but it goes without saying that conditions in the countryside are difficult to assess. We know that in 1582 two rural districts (*herreder*) on the island of Lolland had registered 121 and 194 poor respectively, and given them badges; a number which would have constituted 2.5–3.5 per cent of the local population.[29] Of the 633 biographies recorded by the local minister of the parishes of Sørbymagle and Kirkerup on the island of Zealand between 1646 and 1688, a considerable number were described as poor, but only twenty-nine as beggars, of whom only eighteen were local; in other words less than 3 per cent of the dead the minister buried during that period. The majority were servants who had been dismissed, cripples or children who had been abandoned after the authorities, relations and others, 'had tried to act in their best interest', as the minister wrote in 1685.[30]

Even if we accept the period's definition of the deserving poor it is evident that the authorities only considered those who were experiencing extreme want because of severe physical and mental handicaps, orphans, poor schoolchildren, and the old and infirm as worthy recipients of outdoor relief, if they could not be maintained in the local hospitals. Even if contemporaries did not operate with a minimum level for subsistence the surviving sources indicate that local authorities tried to tackle what they considered temporary or fluctuating poverty through tax reductions or exemptions. Apart from vagrants, whom nobody recognised as deserving of assistance, the authorities clearly distinguished between the long-term deserving poor, who were destitute as a consequence of physical or mental debility, and the short-term poor, who are best described as 'fiscally poor'. This distinction provided the flexibility for the authorities to deal separately with individual cases or take specific initiatives in years of dearth, thus defusing possible social tension.[31]

The surviving sources indicate that tax exemptions and arrears peaked, in the countryside as well as the towns, during the early 1630s, but also that the picture returned surprisingly quickly to what had been the norm, even in war-ravaged Jutland. Widespread impoverishment did, however, not materialise until after 1645, as a consequence of renewed warfare and occupation, and after the taxation had reached record levels (the tax demands grew considerably after the introduction of absolutism in 1660), by which time it was further magnified by an extended economic slump; only the kingdom's larger landowners and wealthier merchants appear to have been able to take advantage of the boom generated by the Thirty Years' War in the years 1629–43. What matters in this context is the marked tendency during the 1630s to try to channel private as well as public funds into the hands of the authorities, while simultaneously introducing a stream of statutes directed against vagrants and vagrancy. By 1636 the government was desperate to stop, or at least minimise the stream of refugees arriving from war-torn Germany, and an order forbidding beggars and vagrants from carrying arms was issued.

Unfortunately, the lack of any detailed research means that we are yet unable to say what forms of piety caused individuals to give alms, donations and gifts for the benefit of the poor in post-Reformation Denmark. Odd reasons for charitable donations can occasionally be found. In 1636 a town councillor in Nakskov donated 100 thalers for the benefit of poor schoolboys, being grateful that 'the murder' of his cat had been solved.[32] Rather tastelessly in 1617, a burgher in Copenhagen made a charitable gift to schoolboys and the poor dependable on his own recovery from an illness.[33] However, such statements remained the exception.

Nearly a century after the Reformation the need for penance and atonement, in spite of their Catholic connotations and the reformers' rejection of good works, remained major imperatives for charitable giving. Thus in 1587 the nobleman Erik Bille of Søholm donated some of his estate to the hospital in Odense in order to soothe his conscience, having committed manslaughter; while in 1616 Christoffer Friis of Farskov left money to the school in Ålborg for similar reasons.[34] A more orthodox justification of a charitable gift was offered in 1631 by a town councillor of Ribe, Mogens Grave, 'being in good health and prospering, to the honour of God the Almighty, the many deserving and helpless poor in Ribe, who are ashamed to knock on people's doors and ask for assistance, for their special relief, benefit, and blessing and for ourselves, next to God's assistance, as an eternal and honest reminder'. The Ribe councillor evidently distrusted the honesty of future trustees and administrators, since he finished his letter of foundation with curses against those who might spend the capital and interest on other purposes.[35]

That piety was the driving force behind charitable initiatives is undoubtedly best illustrated by the activities of the nobleman/theologian Holger Rosenkrantz of Rosenholm. In spite of the difficult economic circumstances in the years 1627–40, he and his wife, Sofie Brahe, spent nearly 8 per cent of their annual income helping poor agricultural workers and providing contributions for charities; and during the years 1628–32 when Jutland was occupied by Imperial troops they increased their charity to nearly 12 per cent; similar charitable contributions were made by their immediate family among the aristocracy on the island of Funen and by their religious associates. This benevolence continued in spite of Rosenkrantz and his allies falling foul of the leaders of the Lutheran Church in the drive for uniformity within the church.[36] It should be emphasised, however, that the circle around Rosenkrantz were not alone in being motivated to charity by piety and godliness, but that such sentiments and actions characterised much of the nobility and many of the leading merchants of the period.

Towards the end of the sixteenth century, a certain reaction against the government's ambition to centralise health care provision and poor relief which had developed after the Reformation, can be seen in the new initiatives to create local hospitals and schools. It is more than likely that developments on the islands of Funen and Lolland from the 1580s were a protest against the tendency by the magistracy in Odense to favour its own inhabitants when admitting new inmates/patients to the diocesan hospital in the former Franciscan monastery. By then gentry and burghers in and around the coastal towns had begun to establish, and financially support, local hospitals and schools, while members of the nobility on Funen had begun creating estate- or parish-hospitals in the countryside. This move was initiated by Niels Friis in the village of Hesselager in 1597, but his example was quickly followed by others, such as Pernille Gyldenstierne of Kærstrup, Ebbe Munk and Sidsel Høeg of Fjellebro (who were all associates of Holger Rosenkrantz) and Jørgen Brahe of Hvedholm.[37]

This trend among the nobility on Funen was subsequently followed in other regions of the country. From the period 1625–48 we know of at least fifteen examples of the creation of new estate- or parish-hospitals and schools. This charity may be seen as patriarchal or necessary initiatives in a period of crisis. It is, however, noteworthy that a number of donors, nobles as well as burghers, retained the right to chose the recipients of their charity during their own lifetime. This was the case of the legacy for seventeen resident poor in Aarhus donated in 1629 by Else Marsvin of Stenalts, and the massive legacy from Anne Friis in 1636.[38] It is more than likely that these examples are representative of a deeper hostility towards growing government control and centralisation.

That the success of the local reforms of charity and poor relief in Copenhagen, Ribe and Odense was only partial does not mean that charitable inclinations decreased when the crisis had been weathered; surviving figures from the voluntary collections in the above towns and in Viborg appear to point in the opposite direction – to an increase in charitable giving.[39] Of greater importance for the assessment of the balance between private and public charity in the period, after the Reformation until the introduction of absolutism in 1660, is the increased importance and significance of donations from private individuals.

The figures in Table 7.1 can only be taken as an indication of the way things were changing, not as precise data. Information about a number of donations have long disappeared, while others were amalgamated over time. The actual distribution of the 584 donations/legacies can provide us with some guidance to the social developments even though we do not yet know the precise amounts.

Table 7.1   Charitable donations for poor relief and education 1536–1660

	Poor relief			Schools			Total
	C	P	I	C	P	I	
1536–60	48	3	2	36	8	0	97
1561–85	24	6	1	39	9	1	80
1586–1610	6	33	0	9	23	1	72
1611–35	11	55	1	10	62	1	140
1636–60	13	79	3	17	82	1	195
Total	102	176	7	111	184	4	584
Percentage							
1536–60	50	3	2	37	8	0	
1561–85	30	7	1	49	11	2	
1586–1610	8	46	0	13	32	1	
1611–35	8	39	1	7	44	1	
1636–60	7	40	1	9	42	1	
Total	17	30	1	19	32	1[40]	

Note: C=Crown; P=Private individuals (noble, eclessiastical, burgher); I=Institutions

The figures confirm the view that the crown fulfilled its obligation and responsibility immediately after the Reformation, assisting in the re-organisation, and helping to finance poor relief, hospitals and schools across the country. These efforts probably met the minimum criteria needed to support the deserving poor; but apart from yet another major effort by the crown during the years of dearth following the end of the Seven Years' War with Sweden in 1570, the period was mainly characterised by the growing intervention against vagrants and sturdy beggars, mainly through the use of forced labour, while the major statute of 1587 finally provided clear and lasting guidelines for the distinction between the deserving and undeserving poor. These coercive measures were supplemented by Christian IV via his attempts to re-socialise the poor, often through mercantilist schemes, such as the House of Correction in 1605 and the Orphanage, and of course his plans for the creation of a general hospital in 1627, modelled on the best European examples.

That the crown's contributions to charity peaked shortly before the statute of 1587 demonstrates that a cohesive government policy was in place in the social domain. It is, however, remarkable that coinciding with this change in government attitude there followed an expansion of private charity evenly shared between burghers, clerics and nobles. A closer analysis of the sources indicates that the greatest increase in private charity took place around the turn of the sixteenth century, and that the stream of private donations peaked towards the end of Christian IV's reign. Taking into consideration a delay of between one and two decades, this corresponds closely with similar developments in England.

It is probably too early to try to determine the religious, ideological and material rationale for this increase in private charity. In the case of England, the growing wealth of aristocracy and merchants was significant, as was the deep economic crisis of the 1590s which necessitated action in order to preserve law and order. Likewise, in Denmark the increased wealth of the dominant groups in society, such as prominent merchants and aristocracy, may well, to some extent, explain the expansion in private charity; whereas its possible connections to the increased orthodoxy of the Lutheran Church are difficult to determine.[41] What remains is the fact that the increase in private charity coincided with the new initiatives of Christian IV. That private charity peaked during the last years of the king's reign, which was characterised by crisis and conflict, is not surprising. The prevailing feeling at the time, namely that the Day of Judgement was imminent, can only have served to enhance the drive towards charity.

However, it cannot be claimed that the private and public initiatives of the 1630s to tackle the poverty brought about by war and crisis represented a turning point. Basically, the government did little more than expand and refine already existing guidelines, narrowing the definition of the deserving poor and prohibiting begging, while encouraging local authorities to hunt down sturdy beggars. The situation remained unchanged under later governments in the absolutist era; their hands remained tied, partly because they felt obliged to concentrate resources and energy on rebuilding the country after the wars with Sweden, and partly because the governments did not possess the necessary local and central administration needed for this task. Instead they were forced to leave poor relief, like so many other 'public' tasks, to the local nobility and gentry. Thus it was not until Frederik IV's reign and his poor law of 1708 that the most pressing shortcomings were finally amended and new guidelines provided, but even then much of what was instituted had firm roots in the past.

Nevertheless, the reforms of poor relief in the 1630s are of great importance. Admittedly, compared with the ambitions which the young king, Christian IV, had expressed at the beginning of his reign, they did not seek to achieve the same wide-ranging, centralising and mercantilist goals. But like the fundamental order for ecclesiastical discipline of 1629, the initiatives in the 1630s had similar consequences: the responsibility for the administration of poor relief and social control came to rest firmly in the hands of the local lay and ecclesiastical authorities, supervised within each diocese by the royal administrator and the bishop. In this respect Christian IV's initiatives represent new traits which match the developments in other areas, such as growing administrative centralisation, professionalisation and control; together these developments portend the emergence of the modern state, even if government or public responsibility for social welfare remained a long way off.

NOTES

1 O. Nielsen, *Kjøbenhavns Historie og Beskrivelse*, IV, Copenhagen 1885, 18.

2 H. Johannsen, *Den ydmyge konge. Kirkens Bygning og Brug*, Studier tilegnet Elna Møller, Copenhagen 1983, 127–54.

3 V. A. Secher (ed.) *Corpus constitutionum Daniæ*, IV, Copenhagen 1897, nos 99 and 192; see also K. Erslev, *Aktstykker og Oplysninger til Rigsraadets og Stændermødernes Historie*, I, Copenhagen 1883–85, 365 ff., 384 ff.

4 *Corpus constitutionum*, IV, no. 310; see also *Kancelliets Brevbøger 1627–9*, Copenhagen 1927, 116, 176, 183 ff., 479, 785. Characteristic examples of this general mood can be seen from the responses of Councillor Jacob Ulfeld in 1627 and the burghers in the towns of Jutland in 1629; Erslev, *Aktstykker og Oplysninger*, I, 66 ff., 204 ff., 209; for the statute of 1629 enforcing church discipline, see *Corpus constitutionum*, IV, 448–50.

5 J. Bossy, 'The Social History of Confession in the Age of the Reformation', *Transactions of the Royal Historical Society*, 5th series, XXV, 1975, 21–38

6 See R. Bireley, *Religion and Politics in the Age of the Counterreformation*, Chapel Hill NC, 1981.

7 F. V. Mansa, *Bidrag til Folkesygdommenes og Sundhedsplejens Historie i Danmark*, Copenhagen 1873, 294–307.

8 O. Nielsen (ed.) *Kjøbenhavns Diplomatarium*, V, nos 192, 103, Copenhagen 1882, see also *Kancelliets Brevbøger 1627–9*, 44.

9 See B. Tierney, *Comparative Studies in Society and History*, I, The Hague 1958–9, 360–82; for what follows see J.-P. Gutton, *La Société et les Pauvres en Europe*, Paris 1974; and B. Pullan, 'Catholics and the Poor in Early Modern Europe', *Transactions of the Royal Historical Society*, 5th series, XXVI, 1976, 15–34.

10 See T. Riis (ed.) *Aspects of Poverty in Early Modern Europe*, II, Odense 1986, 218 ff.

11 See D. C. Coleman, *Labour in the English Economy in the Seventeenth Century: essays in economic history*, II, ed. E. M. Carus-Wilson, London 1962, 296–98.

12 See P. Slack, *Poverty and Policy in Tudor and Stuart England*, London 1988; and Chapter 11 of this volume.

13 T. Dahlerup, 'Den Sociale Forsorg og Reformationen i Danmark', *Historie*, new series, XIII, 1979–80, 194–207; see also M. H. Nielsen, *Fattigvæsenet i Danmark 1536–1708* (Årbog for Dansk Kulturhistorie), Copenhagen 1897, 69–124.

14 *Danske Samlinger*, VI, 1870–1, 346.

15 O. Olsen, *Christian IVs Tugt- og Børnehus*, 2nd ed., Aarhus 1978.

16 H. Sejerholt, 'Omsorgen for de Fattige', *Aarhus gennem Tiderne*, II, eds J. Clausen *et al.*, Aarhus 1940, 350.

17 E. Ladewig Petersen, *Dansk Social Historie*, 3, Copenhagen 1980, 352–5; see also Coleman, *Labour in the English Economy*, 291 ff.

18 See Chapter 3 of this volume.

19 Erslev, *Aktstykker og Oplysninger*, II, Copenhagen 1887–8, 202.
20 *Corpus Constitutionum*, IV, no. 336; and *Kjøbenhavns Diplomatarium*, II, Copenhagen 1874, 786 ff. That the king's initiative was recent and caused by the growing social deprivation can be seen from the fact that Christian IV as late as 1627 had hoped to see the 'silkhouse' reopened and continued. See C. F. Bricka and J. A. Fridericia (eds) *Kong Christian den Fjerdes egenhændige Breve 1589–1648*, II, Copenhagen 1969 (reprint), no. 57.
21 *Kjøbenhavns Diplomatarium*, V, 115; see also 117 ff. By March 1630 the king was still urging the committee to accelerate its work; see the statute of 8 March 1630, *ibid.*, VI, 206–8, *Corpus Constitutionum*, IV, no. 539; and M. Rubin, *Tabellarisk Fremstilling af Kjøbenhavns Fattigvæsen i Tidsrummet 1816–78* (Tabelværk til Kjøbenhavns Statistik no. 4), Copenhagen 1879, 9–12; and Nielsen, *Kjøbenhavns Historie*, IV, 15–23.
22 M. R. Ursin, *Stiftsstaden Viborg*, Copenhagen 1849, 243.
23 J. Kinch, *Ribe Bys Historie og Beskrivelse*, II, Odder 1884, 328–31, 773–83; O. Degn, *Rig og Fattig i Ribe*, I, Aarhus 1981, 365 ff.; *Fra Ribe Amt*, XXII, no. 2 (1982), 360 ff.
24 See T. Kaarsted *et al.* (eds) *Odense bys Historie*, II, Odense 1984, 395–411.
25 Ladewig Petersen, *Dansk Social Historie*, III, 102–11.
26 H. P. Mumme, *Bidrag til Odense Byes Historie*, Odense 1857, 61–7
27 Degn, *Rig og Fattig*, I, 42, 45, 54, 367.
28 M. R. Ursin, *Viborg*, Copenhagen 1849, 243 ff.; and P. F. Edvardsen, *Schielschiør Købsteds nuværende og fortidige Tilstand*, Skelskør 1759, 583–90.
29 C. Thorsen, in *Arkiv og Museum*, V (1913), 244–6; and H. Matthiesen, in *ibid.*, 2nd series, I (1917), 113.
30 See O. Højrup (ed.) *Levnedsløb i Sørbymagle og Kirkerup kirkebøger 1646–1731*, I–II, Copenhagen 1963–8.
31 See Riis, *Aspects of Poverty*, II, 217 ff.
32 H. de Hofman, *Samlinger af Publique og Private Stiftelser, Fundationer og Gavebreve*, I–XI, 1755–80, see XI, 109 ff.
33 *ibid.*, X, 280.
34 *ibid.*, VI, 289 ff., IV, 128 ff.
35 *ibid.*, V, 506 ff.; see also Kinch, *Ribe Bys Historie*, II, 342 ff.
36 H. Paulsen, *Sophie Brahes Regnskabsbog 1627–40*, Viborg 1955; see also the review of this work by E. Ladewig Petersen, in *Historisk Tidsskrift*, series 11, IV (1953–6), 663.
37 Kaarsted, *Odense by*, II, 202–4.
38 Hofman, *Samlinger*, II, 134–6; see also Sejerholt, *Omsorgen*, 347 ff.
39 Kaarsted, *Odense by*, II, 408 ff.; *Fra Ribe amt*, XXII, 360 ff.
40 The figures in Table 7.1 have been collated from *Regesta Diplomatica Historicæ Danicæ*, I–II, Det kgl. danske Videnskabernes Selskab, Copenhagen 1847–1907. Only around three-quarters of the donations found here have been noted by H. de Hofman, *Samlinger*. Hofman, however, did not include charitable legacies in Scania.

Futhermore, the actual definition of what constitutes a legacy is often problematic.

41 We know of legacies/donations from only two peasants, both for parish schools in 1617 and 1646 respectively; see Hofman, *Samlinger*, V, 377 ff., and VII, 313. For charity in England, see W. K. Jordan, *Philanthropy in England 1480–1660*, London 1959; and C. Wilson, 'Poverty and Philanthrophy in Early Modern England', in T. Riis (ed) *Aspects of Poverty in Early Modern Europe*, Florence 1981, 253–79.

Chapter 8

Health care and poor relief in Sweden and Finland
c. 1500–1700

E. I. Kouri

Reminders of social norms which were in force during an earlier pagan period can be found in Nordic regional medieval legislation (*landskapslagarna*). They demonstrate that the care of the sick and poor before the arrival of Christianity rested with the extended family. Within pagan society the family played a prominent part, and it was not until the beginning of the early modern period that the importance of the family began to decline in the legislation. From the later Middle Ages Finland had gradually been drawn into the Swedish sphere of influence and Swedish regional legislation was slowly being adapted.

The universal influence of the medieval Catholic Church can be traced in the regional laws of Scandinavia, which placed responsibility for poor relief on the tax-paying peasantry. Of the tithe payable to the church, a part was retained for the poor. The distribution of this share of the tithe intended for the poor rested with the peasants. However, we do not know whether this practice was adopted in Finland. On the other hand, we can safely assume that the regional legislation did not introduce any fundamental changes to the way the sick and poor were cared for.[1]

The impact of Catholic teaching and the developments in the urban centres of Europe began to affect the towns of Sweden and Finland by the later Middle Ages. The relief of poverty gradually came to be seen as contributing towards the salvation of the donor's soul. In the mercantile centres of Europe the distribution of charity became a large-scale enterprise, which received the attention of the church and the magistracy as well as individuals. Medieval theologians were not totally blind to social realities. Even if voluntary poverty was praised as a particular Christian virtue, the attitude of the church to the urban poor, and vagrant beggars in particular, was characterised by suspicion; and the destabilising effects of poverty were condemned.[2]

Hostelries for pilgrims and institutional care for the sick had been provided by monasteries during the Middle Ages. Their most common form was the *xenodocium* (hostel), often described as a hospital. These hostels/hospitals were the original centres for the distribution of indoor as well as outdoor relief for travellers and the poor. When poor relief was gradually centralised in the towns during the fourteenth and fifteenth centuries, the significance of these institutions increased. Out of them grew a system of poor relief centred around the poorhouse. The creation of this type of institution in Sweden is closely connected with the spread of leprosy in Scandinavia. In order to isolate lepers, houses dedicated to St Giles (*St Göran*) were erected outside the walls of many towns. Within the boundaries of present-day Sweden, twenty-four hospitals for lepers existed during the Middle Ages. Meanwhile, a number of houses of the Holy Spirit were refounded in order to give shelter and food to the destitute. At the start of the fourteenth century, houses of the Holy Spirit already existed in Stockholm, Uppsala, Visby and Kalmar. They were financed partly from taxation, partly from private donations. Involved in their day-to-day running were representatives of the crown as well as members of the local magistracies.[3]

Similar developments took place in Finland. The monasteries offered some assistance to the poor, but in Åbo a hospital dedicated to St Giles had already come into existence in 1355, as had a house dedicated to the Holy Spirit which by 1396 had been expanded to incorporate a special ward for lepers. Legally these institutions were the responsibility of the chapter of the cathedral in Åbo; financially, however, they were dependant on local taxes. In Viborg a house of the Holy Spirit is mentioned for the first time in 1445 and a hospital dedicated to St Mary Magdalene is referred to in 1475. This hospital, which catered for lepers from most of eastern Finland, owned considerable estates, but was partly financed through a leper tax collected in the fiefs of Viborg, Borgå and Tavstehus. All these institutions, however, were comparatively modest in both scale and effectiveness.[4]

During the Middle Ages disease was generally considered to result from sins and the church was more often than not uninterested in medical care. Instead, it worked through exorcism, prayer and blessings. According to the missal manuscript preserved for the house of the Holy Spirit in Stockholm a greater number of holy days and holy communions were celebrated here than was otherwise the norm for the diocese. Certain saints carried special significance for the sick and the poor and each institution tended to have its own patron saint. In Åbo they prayed to Mary the Blessed Virgin, St Giles, St Gertrude and the first bishop of Åbo to suffer martyrdom, the English-born St Henry (the national saint of Finland).[5]

At the time of the Reformation and the complex political changes known as the emergence of the nation state, the Catholic institutions which had looked after the sick and the poor were faced with fundamental changes. While territorial governments sought to bring what had been an international church under their control, they also used the opportunity to take charge of the local charitable institutions.[6] This was a process which went far from smoothly. It often proved easier to demolish the medieval Catholic institutions which had encouraged charity towards the less fortunate and provided relief for them than to re-create these institutions in a reformed community. Even if neighbourly love and charity was formalised and often made compulsory, the public attitude towards poverty and the poor retained many of its medieval features, although new elements were added.

The Reformation constitutes a watershed in the history of health care provision and poor relief in the kingdom of Sweden and Finland. Many charitable Catholic institutions were already faced with serious economic difficulties before the Reformation – especially those belonging to the mendicant orders. According to canon law they should either have amalgamated with or have been taken over by their nearest sister-institutions; instead they became a prime target for the reformers. Since the crown after the Reformation portrayed itself as God's representative on earth, thus justifying its sequestration of most of the estates and income belonging to the Catholic Church, it might be expected that these charitable, Catholic institutions would be included in the crown's takeover which began in 1527. That, however, was not the case. Gustav Vasa specifically excluded and protected these institutions. Repeatedly the king intervened to protect houses of the Holy Spirit and hospitals from the encroachment of private individuals, pointing out that these institutions should all be preserved for the benefit of the kingdom's sick and poor. Thus they continued to honour the promises made to donors of an earlier period, even if the spiritual dimension such as regular prayers and vigils for the souls of the donors had now stopped. Likewise, in the case of a number of hospitals in Götaland, Gustav Vasa intervened to make sure that they would retain the traditional 'spital-part' of the tithe or be compensated by a similar amount. This, however, was far from enough to secure these institutions financially and they regularly needed extra funds from crown lands, while private donations continued to pay for most of their needs.[7]

Hospitals did not depend solely on the crown for their public funding; nearly half came from the local parishes. Despite their laicisation these institutions did not lose their ecclesiastical character altogether after the Reformation. They retained their own chaplains and maintained regular services on a daily basis with grace being said before meals. Similarly the election of supervisors, which was conducted by burgomasters and town councillors, had to be sanctioned by the local bishop and clergy. The supervisors were responsible for the care of the patients and the finances of the institutions they presided over. Furthermore, in the wake of the Reformation a centralisation of these charitable institutions, encouraged by general social and economic trends, took place within most towns.

After the Reformation a series of statutes, ordinances, decrees and bills were promulgated to regulate the care of the poor, the sick and the elderly. They reflect not only the way the Swedish and Finnish authorities viewed the poor who depended on charity, but also the religious, social and political rationale behind the structure and organisation of care and relief. In this context developments relating to health care provision in Stockholm proved significant for the realm as a whole. In September 1533 the magistracy passed a statute for the hospital and house of the Holy Spirit, which was to set the pattern for other hospitals in the realm – not least because it received the king's approval. Västerås became the first town to follow the example of Stockholm. For more than a generation, from 1533 until the 1560s, this hospital statute regulated the affairs of Swedish and Finnish hospitals.[8]

According to the statute of 1533, the poor who were to be hospitalised had to be so ill that they were unable to look after themselves. If they had property and money these possessions were to be offered to any relations willing and able to look after them. If their family and friends refused to care for them, they were to lose all chance of any future inheritance, which presumably went to the hospital where they received care. The Stockholm statute specified that only the resident poor were to be accepted by the hospitals. The sick and destitute originating from the surrounding villages were to be returned to their localities where they were to be looked after by the local parish. Furthermore, in the statutes relating to Stockholm and Västerås, begging was prohibited, drunkenness punished, and the able-bodied poor forced to work in return for the alms they received. Cleanliness was encouraged since the statutes emphasised that the poor were to bath regularly. Compared with the statute for the medieval hospital in Enköping, the rules of 1533 had become tougher and more comprehensive. The patients or inmates were no longer left to their own devices, but were closely supervised. Besides the supervisors, who were to be godly men, an administrator (*syssloman*) who 'loved the poor and would live and die together with them in the hospital, if such a man could be found' was to be appointed.[9] This statement indicates that the administrator was supposed to look after the interests of the residents if need arose. In the case of Stockholm it was emphasised that a physician should be appointed to attend residents.

With the approval of the burgomasters and councillors, 'free brethren', i.e. paying pensioners, could be accepted by the hospital in Stockholm. These residents were mainly recruited from among the better off citizens who, due to age and health, were unable to look after themselves. On their death, these 'free brethren' were to leave their possessions to the hospital which had cared for them. They appear to have been given a separate section of the hospital for their accommodation and meals, the so-called *konventsstuga* (common room). Around 1557 the hospital housed twenty-four 'free brethren', while eleven residents were housed in the 'spital room', two were placed in the 'bath-room' and no less than sixty-one in the 'sick room'. In this latter group we also find a number of mentally ill.[10]

In the years before the parliament (*Riksdag*) of Västerås, which met in 1527, there were six institutions concerned with health care provision and poor relief in Stockholm, all controlled by the burgomasters and the council: the house of the Holy Spirit, St Giles' Hospital, All Souls Court (*Själagården*), the Sunday Charity, the Friday Charity and a chamber for the sick. After the Reformation, from 1531, the city's main hospital was situated in the former Franciscan monastery on Gråmunkeholmen (today's Riddarholmen). In 1558 it was moved to Danviken for 'hygienic reasons'. In 1561 this hospital housed sixty-one inmates/patients in its north wing, and sixty-three people were cared for in the south wing. Furthermore, the south wing had a special section for lepers, including those suffering from the pox, containing sixteen patients. Another twenty residents should, however, be added to this number. They were 'pensioners' who paid a fee for board and lodging.

According to the accounts for 1567, Danviken Hospital received its income from a number of sources. Among them were annual payments from 'the poor peasants in Duvnäs, Skuru and Järla'; regular payments from farms in Sickla and Hammarby, donations from wills, and part of the tithes collected by some royal bailiffs. By far the greatest contribution, however, came from the offerings collected at the services in Stockholm – no less than 2,347 marks – of which the greatest single contributor was the king with 200 marks.[11]

It is significant that the statute of 1533 for the hospital and the house of the Holy Spirit in Stockholm were drawn up by the leading Swedish religious reformer Olaus Petri, in collaboration with the magistracy in Stockholm. It was, in other words, a restructuring closely linked to the Reformation. As such these institutions were to serve the Christian community of Stockholm by offering care and relief to the destitute and sick. True Christian charity, as a consequence of faith and grace, was to be the basis for this charity. Gone was the doctrine of good works which, with the assistance of the Catholic Church, might ease a donor's way to salvation. The fact that a chaplain was attached to the hospital to catechise the inmates/ patients in the new Protestant faith further underlines this statute's roots in Reformation theology. However, popular religious attitudes did not change overnight in Sweden or elsewhere, and the personal reward motive continued to play a significant part in Protestant charity throughout the early modern period. But it is noteworthy that it came to be used differently by Protestants. Where late medieval Catholic charity was performed with the certainty of reward in the afterlife, being a claim already underwritten by the church, Protestant donors could rely on no such guarantees and could only nurture a pious hope of reward.[12]

Undoubtedly, the sick and poor admitted to the hospital in Stockholm were made aware of their dependance on the benevolence of lay, as well as the new ecclesiastical, authorities. However, it was emphasised in the statutes that they were to be treated leniently. Depending on whether those who transgressed the rules of the hospital were 'free brethren and sisters' paying for their keep or poor inmates, the punishment incurred varied significantly. That they were far more detailed and punitive for the pensioners, who paid for their lodging, is hardly surprising. Chances of rebellion against the strict rules and discipline of the hospital by those who did not depend on public charity exclusively must have been much greater. They, after all, had a choice and might be able to get by in the outside world, whereas expulsion of those poor and sick who depended wholly on public charity would have had devastating consequences for such individuals.[13]

The Swedish reform of health care provision and poor relief was imitated in Finland. In Åbo the hospital (for lepers only) and the house of the Holy Spirit were unified and brought under the same management. From then on, the country was served by two centralised hospitals placed in Åbo and Viborg respectively, where they were under diocesan administration. We know that the hospital in Åbo had around forty lepers among its inmates/patients in 1570, while the number of lepers in Viborg was around half that. Apart from these two centralised institutions, a small hospital came into existence in Helsinki, attached to the royal residence, which was later financed by the crown. Despite support from King Johan III, attempts to create a small hospital/sick chamber in Borgå proved unsuccessful.[14]

The hospitals in Finland mainly cared for those who suffered from leprosy, epidemic diseases and the pox, while room was also found for a fair number of mentally ill. Certain social groups, such as ministers and their families, seem to have enjoyed privileged access to these institutions, while other groups in the post-Reformation era, such as the elderly and poor, found that their chance of being admitted had diminished. Thus the Finnish hospitals played only a marginal role in providing poor relief. The changes experienced by the Finnish hospital in the sixteenth and seventeenth centuries can be considered a first step in a development which eventually served to separate health care from poor relief.[15]

In 1544 a parliament was summoned to deal with the emergency brought about by the recent popular revolt in southern Sweden. It had been caused mainly by social and economic grievances, but the remaining Catholic clergy had encouraged the rebels. This incident convinced Gustav Vasa that a complete break with Catholicism was now in the interests of the crown.[16] He re-intensified the crown's sequestration of ecclesiastical property and income. The Swedish Church, however, was allowed to retain part of the traditional tithe, some of which was supposed to finance hospitals from the middle of the sixteenth century onwards: the towns including their hospitals remained under royal protection. Financially, however, the hospitals depended on occasional assistance to keep them going. This was a system, or lack of one, which meant that they regularly found themselves short of capital. The supervisor was responsible for providing for the patients while keeping an eye on the hospital's economy in general. When a hospital experienced financial difficulties the supervisor normally approached the king in order to secure an admonition of the clergy to help find the necessary funds. Thus during the sixteenth century a development took place which increasingly brought the hospitals under the influence of the crown. Occasionally, in the reign of Gustav Vasa, the royal treasury inspected the accounts of hospitals. This practice seems to have become the rule in the reign of his son, Erik XIV (1560–8).[17]

According to the statutes of most towns, it fell to the children to care for their elderly, sick or handicapped parents. In cases where there were no children, or they were unable to fulfill their obligations, other relatives were expected to take their place. If these relatives refused to honour their obligations they were to be excluded from receiving any inheritance. Thus, in the first place, social solidarity was restricted to the nuclear family and only when that avenue had been exhausted did it incorporate the extended family. It was within this context that the problems associated with old age and disease were to be tackled. However, in post-Reformation Sweden, other possibilities of social protection and assistance were available to those who were not destitute. Childless couples could, apart from the obligatory half of the estate, bequeath each other 'third penny' (*tredje penning*) which meant that they were entitled to a third of the rest of the estate. This arrangement was supposed to insure them against possible future claims on them by elderly or sick relatives. Another avenue was open to those who had some possessions and estate, but lacked relatives and were unable to look after themselves. They could make private arrangements similar to those who became 'free brethren and sisters' in the hospital, without necessarily relinquishing control over all their estate.[18]

Other forms of social security were obtainable for merchants and craftsmen through membership of corporations and guilds. In Stockholm such organisations might be established along cultural and ethnic lines, serving the need of the resident German and Finnish communities exclusively. Even the crown tried to provide some care for its employees. It demonstrated particular concern for old soldiers and prisoners of war held abroad. In the 1560s instructions were issued to royal administrators to make sure that sick and elderly soldiers who had served in the local castles were offered free food and beer until their death. When, during the mid-1560s, a serious outbreak of plague badly affected the Swedish navy in Stockholm, a new military hospital was created on Gråmunkeholmen. Those soldiers, however, who suffered from the pox, were transferred to the newly founded hospital in Danviken, where they were treated in the leprosy wing.[19]

The strengthening of royal power from the middle of the sixteenth century, which accompanied the rapid growth of central administration, together with the transformation of Swedish society from a feudal to an estate-based kingdom, had significant implications for the country's labour policy and the closely connected ideas about poor relief and health care provision. The general demographic development in early modern Europe provides a backdrop for these changes. In Scandinavia as in most of Europe, excluding Finland, the population grew rapidly during the sixteenth century, while continuing to expand at a much slower pace during the seventeenth century. This population growth resulted in rising food prices which were accompanied by falling real wages for workers in most of the urban centres of Europe, including Sweden. The result was a dramatic increase in the number of poor and vagabonds looking for employment.

This coincided with the period when the government expanded its bureaucracy, while demonstrating an active interest in utilising the expanding labour force to promote state initiatives and projects. Thus new developments took place within European social policy during the sixteenth century which were religiously as well as economically and politically inspired, and which were to have considerable implications for future developments in this domain. In accordance with the general trend in Europe towards the end of the sixteenth century, the Swedish government took a tougher stance with regard to the rights, or rather the lack of rights, for servants and farm labourers.[20]

Traditionally, begging had been one of the pillars of poor relief. It was acknowledged that the destitute and invalid were forced to rely on begging for their survival. Even during normal years begging was widespread, while after harvest failures it became endemic. Repeated crop failure often meant that copyholders and smaller farmers were forced to eat their seed corn in order to survive, in which case little or nothing was left for charity. Crises like these had a disastrous effect on the more vulnerable members of society, such as the elderly poor, orphans, the chronically ill and the blind. Their sufferings were recognised by the legislators who repeatedly tried to tackle the problems.

From the late Middle Ages, the authorities had tried to prevent and regulate begging and to set the workshy to work. The Reformation, however, saw an intensification of such state initiatives as were intended to prevent vagrancy and the undeserving poor from receiving alms. Thus the royal administrators did their best to prevent begging in accordance with the decision of the parliament of Västerås in 1527. In Sweden, where the Protestant Church was firmly under royal control, it proved unproblematic to get the church to support such policies.[21] But it should not be forgotten that begging, an act strongly associated in popular Protestant imagination with the excesses of the Catholic Church and the mendicant orders, was considered an activity which ought not to be necessary in a properly organised Christian community built on neighbourly love and Christian charity.

The Reformation century witnessed a transformation in the way the poor and poor relief were perceived in Sweden and Finland. According to medieval Catholicism, poverty was a holy state which served as a reminder to the more fortunate citizens of God and his church, offering them an avenue to salvation by actively showing their charity to the poor and sick. The holiest of the poor were undoubtedly the mendicants – the voluntary poor who had taken orders – who offered the donor the best and safest avenue to salvation or avoidance of purgatory. Whereas inmates/patients in medieval hospitals were expected to pray for the souls of their benefactors, the discipline they lived under appears to have been far from rigorous. This changed dramatically in the sixteenth century, when the poor were constantly reminded of their dependency on charity. They were expected to show their humility and gratitude to the authorities and their benefactors in their daily prayers. That they received charity should not lead them to forget their calling and obligation to look after themselves. It was the intention that the relief they received was to be temporary and serve to help them once more to become active and useful members of the Christian commonwealth. Whereas Catholic charity in the Middle Ages had focused on the benefit to the donor in terms of the afterlife and salvation, and demonstrated little concern for whether the charity offered really benefited the recipients, post-Reformation society of the sixteenth century placed increased emphasis on the distinction between the deserving and the undeserving poor. The former were to be the focus of true Christian charity while the latter, if possible, were to be eradicated. This change in emphasis may well have had more to do with the rejection of the voluntary poor as proper objects for charity by the reformers rather than the emergence of a new Protestant work ethic, which underlined the Christian individual's obligation to work for their keep, as indicated by a number of scholars.[22] These clerical voluntary poor were, after all, a human invention, as opposed to the involuntary poor who were part of the natural world created by God.

The reformers, via their doctrine of 'the priesthood of all believers', had handed back the church to the laity by redefining it as incorporating the whole Christian community with no qualitative difference between clergy and laity. Within this reconstituted Christian community, charity was seen as a way to help the deserving poor regain their position within the local community, while those poor, the undeserving, who refused to take any social responsibility by refusing to work for their upkeep, were to be excluded from the Christian community and receive little or no help.[23]

This change of attitude to and religious view of the poor gradually resulted in them, especially those labelled undeserving, being seen as a threat to society. As such they had to be dealt with by the authorities and were no longer considered a proper object for charity. The governments of late sixteenth-century and early seventeenth-century Sweden came to see the growing number of poor first as a threat to public order and only second as a proper target for public charity. Clearly, it was the growing number of unemployed vagrants and criminals which caught the eye of the authorities, while the respectable poor quietly stuck in deep poverty were often forgotten. Occasionally the government would resort to forced migration or internal deportation to rid certain urban localities of the many rootless vagrants and masterless men they had attracted. A decree of 1546 ordered such 'useless' people to remove themselves to those parts of the countryside from where they originated.[24]

It was those sectors of the population who lived at the margins of society, such as the dispossessed poor in the countryside and the casual labour force in the towns, who suffered most from the new regulations and laws against vagrancy which also dealt with issues such as enforced service for servants and social safeguards in general. Where medieval Swedish regional legislation had defined a beggar as a person who was unable to pay taxes and who was without a permanent residence or permanent work, the laws of the 1540s intensified the pressure on the dispossessed by emphasising that those servants who had neither work nor income were obliged to find service if they were not to be treated as vagrants. Bearing in mind Sweden's expansive foreign policy in the Baltic during the second half of the sixteenth century, the crown evidently had a growing need for soldiers, building workers and other personnel necessary for the armament and military provisions of the kingdom. Consequently it was in the crown's interest that the laws against vagrancy were rigorously enforced.[25]

Noble as well as non-noble landlords developed the concept of lay protection or patronage during this period. In Sweden this found its earliest expression in the aristocratic privileges issued in 1569. This concept was, of course, rooted in the landlords' interest in making sure that the necessary workforce was available for their estates. In the first instance it had developed as a protection against conscription by the crown, but gradually it had become a weapon against the growing problem of vagrancy. Besides men above the age of fifteen this legislation against vagrancy was also directed against women. Initially women might escape by paying a fine, but when caught out repeatedly they were in danger of being incarcerated in workhouses and spinning houses.

The increased shortage of labour in the countryside in the first decades of the seventeenth century, brought about by the growing migration towards the provincial urban centres, often worked to the advantage of the dispossessed. Since most farms in Finland in particular were too small to be able to afford hired workers, children from such families tended to stay and work on family land, thus being prevented from running into trouble with the authorities over vagrancy.[26]

The cumulative effects of increased poverty, disease and invalidity were not personal calamities solely, but affected the whole fabric of society. In tackling these problems the family remained the first port of call, while within the urban communities the craft guilds carried some of the social burden. Under such circumstances those living on the margins of society or those who had left their native communities were exposed. While attempting to create a centralised poor relief system in the towns, the authorities were faced with the additional pressure generated by the increased migration from rural areas towards urban centres. To try and exclude the non-resident poor from assistance was an obvious way of protecting a new and fragile system of poor relief from being overburdened. The wars, harvest failures and general impoverishment of the period caused a futher reduction in an already shrinking rural population and the number of vagrants grew considerably. This process gathered further pace during the period of war between Sweden-Finland and Russia which began in the 1570s. It resulted in increased taxation plus the obligation of the peasantry to provide shelter and board for a growing number of soldiers. This increased burden on the peasantry caused severe hardship: many peasants found it difficult to pay their taxes, fell into debt and eventually lost their farms. The example of the east Finnish province of Savo shows that, of the farms which paid taxes in 1571, only 30 per cent were able to contribute sixteen years later. The farmers' inability to meet their tax demands was made even more difficult by a series of failed harvests during the 1570s. The north of Finland was so badly affected that in the wealthy parish of Kemi the number of profitable farms was halved during this decade. Poverty grew and under-nourishment made the population less resistant to epidemics.[27]

Poor relief and health care were organically linked in the early modern period and the church remained the central agency for its administration and distribution in Finland and most parts of Sweden. The local community continued to be responsible for its own poor. In order to secure the necessary funds for the poor box or common chest, collection vessels were placed in most church porches. This relief, however, was far from enough to meet the growing demand. The new Protestant Church taught that charity was a consequence of faith and grace and Christian love of your neighbour, but not a profitable act – good works – which could help save your soul, as was taught by the Catholic Church. This might explain why charitable donations proved insufficient after the Reformation and why the new charitable institutions repeatedly encountered difficulties. Furthermore, if poverty was no longer considered a 'holy state', it was only a natural progression to consider the poor and impoverished to be a potentially dangerous, workshy, anti-social element.[28] The fact, however, that the administrative sources for such institutions are only available after the Reformation and that no comparative medieval material exists, should militate against such a conclusion. Similarly, the increase in poverty and vagrancy might in themselves explain the shortfalls which occurred, rather than the unwillingness of donors to give, due to the lack of supposed personal gain after good works had been rejected by the reformers.

If the Swedish monarchs are anything to go by, then the rejection of the doctrine of good works was of little or no consequence for charitable giving in the realm. They continued the tradition of royal donations and legacies for charitable institutions, but as opposed to their medieval predecessors the Reformation king, Gustav Vasa, and his son Erik XIV no longer donated funds for institutions which served spiritual as well as charitable needs. Their legacies benefited hospitals and indoor and outdoor relief of the poor only. Gustav Vasa left 400 marks in his will for the hospital in Stockholm, while Erik XIV repeatedly donated sums to hospitals and the poor. In 1564 he donated 6,400 marks to be shared among the kingdom's twenty-one hospitals, and two years later he granted the interest of 10,000 marks to be distributed annually among hospitals, poor households and schools in Sweden.[29]

The obligation of local communities to care for their sick and poor was further emphasised by the government in 1566. The villages were instructed to fulfil their duties and not to encourage their poor to seek support in neighbouring towns where the charitable institutions were already overburdened. Each district was ordered to establish a small infirmary of its own where members of the local community could be cared for. But detailed instructions for the care and relief of the sick and poor in Sweden and Finland were not issued until a Protestant church order finally appeared in 1571. Drafted by Archbishop Laurentius Petri, it was inspired by a number of earlier German Protestant church orders.[30]

The church order stated that the existing hospitals should be expanded in order that each diocesan centre could possess a hospital with at least thirty beds. The administrators were to be elected by the burgomasters in conjunction with the parish clergy and the bishop. With regard to the hospital in Stockholm, it was decided that apart from the royal administrator and the town's most prominent minister, the board should include one of the burgo-masters and two of the councillors. The hospital was commissioned to send out special collectors to all parishes in the diocese equipped with letters of recommendation from the bishop. The local ministers were then expected to recommend these collectors and their cause to their congregations, encouraging their parishioners to give generously. Even if the need for the local communities to support the larger hospitals in the major towns was emphasised in the church order, the local needs were not ignored. It was recommended that each parish establish a small 'sick chamber' or infirmary with room for four to six patients/inmates. Such 'charity rooms' were often established in buildings adjacent to the local churches where regular collections for these institutions were expected to take place. The poor box which was thus established was supposed to be administered separately from other church funds. The church order's specific instructions for the care of elderly ministers, however, continued in the main a medieval Catholic practice.[31]

Evidently, it proved difficult to achieve the ambitious targets set out in the church order of 1571. The expectation that local communities could finance the costs of these reforms, especially after the crown had confiscated most of the wealth of the Catholic Church, often proved unrealistic. Despite these problems, infirmaries were established in many parishes. Thus in east Finland half-a-dozen 'charity chambers' had been established in connection with the local churches by 1582. In Great-Savo these institutions were commonly described as hospitals. They received financial support from the crown, coming from resources which had previously belonged to the hospital in Viborg. Furthermore, we know that public collections in the localities prescribed in the church order took place in the district of Savo. In other areas, such as south-west Finland, in some parishes, not least those dominated by the nobility, 'charity chambers' or infirmaries had come into existence by the end of the sixteenth century. Generally, however, the creation or building of such small hospitals spread only slowly, since the church order of 1686 re-emphasised the obligation of parishes to build such 'charity chambers'.[32]

During the reign of Erik XIV's brother Johan III (1568–92), the crown provided considerable, if erratic, funding for most hospitals in the realm. The lack of political stability, due to the constant struggle for power between Gustav Vasa's sons and his grandson Sigismund, obviously made it difficult for such institutions to attract royal attention on a continuous basis. Later, during the 1590s and the first couple of decades of the seventeenth century, the high incidence of warfare, harvest failures and epidemics further undermined the hospitals' economic basis, while simultaneously making more people destitute and in need of assistance. In particular, the hospitals' income from tithes and other regular sources appear to have suffered in this period. As a result these institutions found it increasingly difficult to assist the growing number of urban sick and poor whom they were obliged to help. This is evident from the complaints which Duke Karl made about the clergy in 1602, pointing out that although the hospitals were maintained largely through royal contributions, seven people had recently died of starvation in the hospital in Uppsala and people were daily found dying in the streets of Stockholm.[33]

People dying from starvation, however, were not an uncommon phenomenon in the streets of the larger towns and cities, of early modern Europe. In Stockholm the number of recognised poor, those who received poor relief on a regular basis, seems to have constituted around 5–6 per cent of the total population, a similar figure to that of most European cities of this period for which we have data.[34] As in most of these cities, Stockholm's population grew rapidly during these years, from close to 10,000 towards the end of the sixteenth century to about 25,000 around the mid-seventeenth century, reaching 50,000 in the early eighteenth century.

In his will of 1605 Duke Karl, who had succeeded his nephew, the deposed king Sigismund, to the Swedish throne in 1599, suggested some ways of dealing with the increasing number of poor who were unable to receive indoor relief in the hospitals. He suggested that a new layer of hospitals be created between the larger 'state hospitals' such as those in Stockholm and Uppsala, and the 'charity chambers' or infirmaries at parish level. These new medium-sized institutions were to be erected in the provincial or district capitals, where they were to be financed by a percentage of the tithes. However, the king evidently only intended these new hospitals as a supplement to the existing system, which he expressly stated he had no wish to tinker with either locally or centrally.[35]

Swedish legislation of the sixteenth and seventeenth centuries repeatedly emphasised that health care provision and poor relief were the obligation of the local parish. The decision of Örebro in

1617 underlined the duty of each congregation to care for its own poor. In his coronation charter of 1611 Gustavus Adolphus had guaranteed the hospitals' traditional income and sources of support. After the peace with Russia at Stolbova in 1617, which secured Karelia and part of Ingermannland for the realm, a period of peace and tranquility followed which saw the initiation of a number of internal building projects and enterprises. Among the reforms Gustavus Adolphus wanted to undertake was a general re-organisation and rationalisation of poor relief and hospitals. In his suggestions for reforms of 1619, which Gustavus Adolphus requested the clergy to discuss and respond to the following year, the king had pointed out that the growing social problems relating to begging were insoluble until the country's hospitals had been put on a better financial footing. Clearly what Gustavus Adolphus had in mind was an amalgamation of the smaller hospitals in the country in order to create larger and centralised institutions, which were then to receive payments from the parishes in accordance with the number of patients originating from the respective local communities. The clergy, however, initially proved unreceptive to the king's ideas for reforms.[36]

Obviously central government in Sweden and Finland, as in the rest of early modern Europe, was more concerned with those subjects who worked, paid taxes and who might serve as soldiers. During the Reformation period, continuing into the 1560s, central authority strove to define its social obligations. In practice this meant that the responsibility for health care and poor relief rested with the towns and the rural districts. In times of crisis such as harvest failures and war, which impoverished large segments of the population, the problem of responsibility was accentuated. This, combined with the enhanced economic position of the nobility, was to a large extent achieved at the cost of further impoverishment of those sectors of society who already had little or nothing to spare, and served to polarise society further. This, for instance, resulted in the emergence of many large freehold farms in Finland in particular at the beginning of the seventeenth century. This group of wealthy farmers, however, had obtained their wealth at the cost of large numbers of small freeholders who had lost their land and joined the dispossessed.[37]

In spite of the Swedish reformers' emphasis on the obligations of good Christians to love and care for their less fortunate neighbours, individual charity proved unable to cope with the increase in demand during the seventeenth century. Faced with an increasing number of destitute and poor who sought assistance, the reaction in Sweden, as elsewhere in Europe, was increasingly to associate poverty with idleness. It proved difficult to establish the network of parish infirmaries originally envisaged by the government, while the larger institutions in the towns were crowded by applicants. Those who were rejected tried to survive through begging, which developed into a scourge in seventeenth-century Sweden. To remedy this situation, central government felt obliged to legislate. In 1624 an order was issued against the activities of beggars and idlers, while eighteeen years later a comprehensive law dealing with the whole issue of begging was passed. This legislation was re-issued in a revised form in 1698.[38]

Of the Swedish legislation dealing with poverty during this period, the order of 1624 was undoubtedly the most significant. Its objective was to rationalise and make the country's health care provision and poor relief 'system' more effective by amalgamating and enlarging existing hospitals while simultaneously ridding them of those inmates, the majority according to government opinion, who were perceived to be idlers and not truly needy. The order went as far as to forbid begging altogether, but to little effect. What the government considered to be a public order problem, caused by idlers and vagrants who were workshy, was in reality the social consequence of prolonged wars, conscription and increased taxation. Futhermore, the crown intended to provide a solid framework for the reformed social institutions through what amounted to an annual tax.[39]

The order of 1624 underlined the need for control and the obligation of the poor and needy to work in return for the charity they received. Those feigning poverty who were caught were to be put to work immediately, and those who refused were to be incarcerated in workhouses and forced to labour. The parish infirmaries, already established in accordance with the guidelines of the church order of 1571, were to be demolished, able-bodied inmates were to be set to work and the rest to be transferred to the nearest hospital.

Although the order of 1624 was approved by parliament, its drastic measures were never fully implemented. Either it proved too great a task to undertake or the government simply found it too costly in both economic and political terms to attempt to introduce such wide-ranging reforms. Consequently health care provision and poor relief continued to develop in early modern Sweden along the traditional lines. Thus in Stockholm in 1626, Olaus Petri's statute of 1533 was re-issued in a revised form, to which was added a special order dealing with order among the poor male inmates of the hospital. One of the most interesting aspects of this order is its reference to the 'alderman or abbot' who was to function as a first among equals among the poor inmates and keep discipline – a kind of institutional sergeant-major similar to the beggar kings who were appointed from among the outdoor poor in many Scandinavian towns.[40]

The changes introduced in 1626 all sought to protect hospital funds from being misused, maladministered or embezzled by officials as well as inmates, pensioners or the poor. It is undoubtedly right to claim that the revised statute of 1626, including the order concerning the poor, displays a much harsher approach to the poor.[41] But we might add that a similar tough approach towards administrators and officials can be found in the same document. It is not the medieval view of the poor as being an especially blessed estate, however, which was finally discarded in the revised Stockholm statute in 1626, but the views of reformers such as Olaus Petri, who were primarily concerned with the care rather than the control aspect of health care and poor relief.

The bill of 1624 had intended the country's twenty-one hospitals to be amalgamated into eleven larger hospitals which would then cater for around one thousand patients. But nothing came of it. However, the government had greater success with its plans for fees payable on the admission of inmates/patients in order to provide a better financial footing for the hospitals. Two fees depending on the quality of the board – one of sixty thalers (*fogdespisordning*) was clearly geared towards pensioners who could pay for their care and another more modest of just twenty thalers (*svenneordning*) intended for poor inmates – were available. The fees were expected to be met in the first instance by the inmates themselves or their relatives, and only if that proved impossible by their local parish, district or town. Even if this rule proved difficult to enforce in practice, it served to reinforce the traditional view that each local community was responsible for its own poor and sick. The bill also served to make clearer the distinction between deserving and able-bodied poor. The latter group should in future be passed over by the hospitals and dealt with by the local workhouses which the 1624 legislation envisaged for each province. In practice, however, this proved difficult to achieve – as did the projected scheme for annual contributions or taxes to finance this reformed and centralised scheme for poor relief and health care.[42]

It is clear that the existing hospitals in Sweden and Finland were unable to meet the increasing demand by the early seventeenth century. We do not know how many inmates/patients the twenty-one hospitals mentioned in the bill of 1624 could cater for, but we know that the largest of them, the hospital in Stockholm, could house ninety patients around the middle of the sixteenth century. A medium-sized hospital such as that in Västerås held forty patients towards the end of the sixteenth century, a figure which remained stable and was the same in 1630. The total capacity of all the hospitals was probably somewhere between 800 and 900 people, a number which the reforms included in the bill of 1624 would have increased by between 10 and 20 per cent had they been implemented. But it is obvious from these figures that the hospitals played only a minor role in caring for the deserving poor in early modern Sweden and Finland.[43]

In the seventeenth century, when leprosy was gradually disappearing from the rest of Europe, for unknown reasons its incidence grew in Sweden and Finland. The bill of 1624 dedicated a paragraph to describing the obligation of local authorities to establish leper wards or hospitals where the lepers could be kept in isolation in order not to infect other patients or healthy members of the Christian commonwealth.[44] Ideally, the new central hospitals envisaged in the bill of 1624 should have separate wards for diseases which were assumed to be infectious such as leprosy and plague, while the mentally ill were also to be given a separate ward.

In spite of all the shortcomings and misuse of the hospitals described in the 1624 bill, the poor and sick fared considerably better within these institutions than without. That the hospitals received a regular income from property and tithes might have guaranteed that the effects of local harvest failures could be alleviated. This was not to be expected by the majority of the poor and sick, who relied on assistance from parish infirmaries in rural districts or on regular or occasional outdoor relief, not to mention, of course, begging.[45]

The fact that the government found it necessary in 1635 to emphasise the obligation of local communities to effectuate the bill of 1624, and that Queen Christina found it necessary to re-issue it, demonstrates how difficult it proved to put into practice. Only moderate adjustments of what had been practice since the 1530s were eventually made.[46] The hospitals continued unchanged, apart from some tightening of the administrative regulations and the introduction of a stricter regime for inmates. The grand plans for the creation of workhouses and orphanages/childrens hospitals in each district were not implemented. The crown's concern for the care of old and invalid soldiers who had served the regime, a concern which was not shared by the Protestant clergy who considered these people to be some of the worst idlers and vagrants, eventually resulted in the creation, in 1638, of a military hospital in the former monastery in Vadstena.[47]

During the period of confessionalisation, the Protestant clergy in Sweden and Finland continued in the prominent role, especially in the countryside, which they had played in charitable affairs since the Reformation. Continuously, the clergy via their sermons and pamphlets kept reminding lay authority and its servants, from central down to local level, of their obligations towards the sick and poor.[48] Many of their sermons demonstrate a deep social awareness combined with a willingness to criticise lay government. Thus in his preaching manual, the Bishop of Åbo, Ericus Erici Sorolainen, who had graduated from the University of Rostock and who presided over the Finnish Church for more than forty years (1583–1625), condemned the brutal and partly illegal taxation which caused peasants to lose house and home and resort to begging while royal administrators accumulated wealth and erected grand new houses.[49] Even if Ericus Erici depended on German inspiration, his examples are fetched from the abuse and misuse of charitable resources in Finland. Undoubtedly, royal servants in the Finnish provinces had greater possibilities for independent action and for chanelling public funds into their own pockets than had their counterparts within the expanding central administration of the German territorial states.[50]

In his diocesan order of 1628, prepared in accordance with the Swedish Church order of 1571, Isaac Rothovius, Ericus Erici's successor in Åbo, stated that each parish was obliged to create an infirmary for the poor and that the local pastor should prevent them from roaming the countryside begging. In practice, however, begging continued to be tolerated within the local community, especially since infirmaries were not established everywhere. Where they came into existence, the parishioners cared for their 'church poor', providing them with clothes and victuals. Some parishes even established poor chests which provided annual financial assistance to the poor.[51]

Several local orders dealing with social policy were issued in Sweden and Finland during the 1630s. In 1632 Johannes Rudbeckius, who had served Gustavus Adolphus as a court preacher and as the king's personal chaplain, and had been closely involved in government business, drafted new statutes for his diocese of Västerås. They were to play an important part as a model for other similar initiatives. Undoubtedly, for those patients/inmates who were prepared to submit to the discipline of the hospital, to work if requested and to pray daily for the Christian authority who provided for them, the institution offered a reasonably secure existence. The order was divided into twelve paragraphs, of which the first six provide the most comprehensive regulation and description of the tasks and obligations of hospital officials seen in early modern Sweden. Two supervisors had the ultimate authority, while the bishop, the local minister, the royal official and the burgomaster had the right to inspect the institution. The minister was responsible for the spiritual wellbeing of patients/inmates and supervised the resident administrator and the housekeeper/mistress. The administrator alone could put the able-bodied poor to work, the income from which could only benefit the hospital, while it also fell to him to appoint collectors for the hospital, who would tour the diocese gathering funds. Rudbeckius's order tightened the rules and regulations concerning the ways hospitals were run. It proved popular with a number of bishops and was recommended to the two Finnish dioceses of Åbo and Viborg.[52]

The surviving rules and regulations for the hospitals demonstrate the discipline which, according to the authorities, should rule these institutions. Those who fell foul of the regulations were to be punished. In repeated cases of misbehaviour, more often than not caused by the immoderate consumption of aquavit, culprits could be expelled. Increasingly during the period of confessionalisation, life in these institutions took on a religious character. Inmates were obliged to attend services, failing which their meals could be withdrawn. Special services were held for those whose illnesses were perceived to be infectious, such as lepers and plague victims. Among the obligatory devotional events were morning prayers, grace and evensong, when the inmates were expected to pray for the authorities and the hospital's benefactors. Similarly, the inmates were to be regularly catechised. It was the hospital chaplain's duty to celebrate communion regularly, and on separate occasions for the lepers, while, of course, providing comfort and spiritual guidance to the sick and dying. Those who died while confined were buried in the hospital's own graveyard and their belongings became the property of the hospital. Sometimes hospital chaplains also served as supervisors in order to supplement their fairly meagre salaries. By the end of the seventeenth century this practice had become the norm in Sweden.[53]

This religious regimen undoubtedly generated both hostility and false piety among patients/inmates, but there were also those who embraced it wholeheartedly. Thus the chaplain to the hospital in Linköping, in the register of death which he kept, made the following entry under 1679: 'Died on 6 March the blind, old and decrepit Raquel Persdotter, who could sing all the hymns in the hymn book and repeat all the sermons way back, including their texts (the Bible text of the day)'.[54]

Evidently the ambitions expressed in the many surviving statutes and regulations of health care and poor relief often had only limited effect in a vast and sparsely populated country like Sweden-Finland, where the power of central government was necessarily limited, especially in Finland. Undoubtedly the number of dispossessed and destitute grew in Finland, with local variations, during the first half of the seventeenth century. Thus in Finland proper the section of the population who were dispossessed grew to 25 per cent in the 1630s and in Österbotten to around 20 per cent. A large proportion of these people were unable to work due to old age, disease and disability.[55]

In the villages and the countryside poor relief often depended on traditional mutual assistance while the larger farms donated the limited charity available. Occasionally we are given a glimpse of social reality here. In a concluding comment added to his parish's census paper in the 1630s, a pastor from middle Finland made the following statement: 'Here we have many tens of such poor creatures, spent, old, blind and invalid, God's miserable beings, whose names are of no interest to Your Lordships'.[56]

The acknowledgement and recognition by local authorities of some of their own poor, expressed in the category 'church poor', in reality served to recognise legally such poor as deserving within the local community. By including such poor in this category, the leaders of the local rural community had publicly recognised their responsibility for these people and they were regularly supported by the parish poor box. But it proved difficult to get most rural parishes to act beyond such measures. The government's attempt, supported by the leaders of the church, to get each parish to establish a small infirmary, proved to be mainly unsuccessful. Lack of support from the local parish clergy undermined this initiative. But in 1639 some parish clergy, such as those ministers who served the communities in Österbotten, promised the government to do their best in making sure that their parishes provided for the local poor. Despite these promises, little improvement in public charity appears to have taken place since the district's peasants continued to complain of irregular begging.[57]

The idea of infirmaries or poor wards was better suited to relieve poverty in towns, but even here the execution of the government's plans differed widely from the way the crown had envisaged them. The burghers were worried about the prospective cost of such institutions and the prospective inmates considered them to be motivated by the wish to exercise control over them and force them to work. In the smaller towns of Finland the creation of such institutions encountered hostility. Eventually they were only established in the towns of Pori and Vaasa in the 1660s and in Oulu towards the end of the century.

For the hospitals proper more was achieved, even in Finland. The medieval hospitals in Åbo and Viborg continued to operate after the Reformation. However, the spread of leprosy in the realm made the creation of new hospitals imperative. In 1550 the hospital in Helsinki was established, the hospital in Pori came into existence in the second decade of the seventeenth century, Seili hospital in Nauvo in 1622 and Kruunukylä hospital in Österbotten in 1632, while shortlived hospitals were founded on the island of Åland, in Savonlinna and in Kainuu in the vicinity of Kajaani.[58]

Kruunukylä hospital was a typical example of a small hospital in Sweden and Finland. Initially it had twenty-five beds, but the number varied over time. In 1651 it housed fourteen lepers, while in a separate building another twelve inmates lived, who were either blind, epileptic, crippled or other deserving poor. An administrator was in charge of the financial affairs and the day-to-day running of the hospital, while the spiritual wellbeing of the inmates/patients was looked after by the chaplain. Supervision was given by the local minister. In accordance with the poor relief order of 1642, all those who entered this institution were to pay a once-for-all levy of twenty silver thalers. If they were unable to find this sum personally it was to be paid by the applicants' relations or local parish.[59]

With little or no effect the order of 1624 had outlawed begging. Consequently the government made a virtue of neccessity in the poor relief order of 1642 by accepting begging as a proper alternative to public support, but only on condition that it took place in an orderly manner. Only beggars carrying special passes issued by the bishops and rural deans were allowed to beg. This was, of course, done in order to distinguish between the deserving and undeserving poor. If found begging, the latter were to be put in irons and set to forced labour. The comprehensive reform attempt of the 1624 order had been abandoned in 1642. Faced with growing social problems and poverty the government had, by then, resigned itself to little more than a holding operation, trying to regulate begging while placing new demands on local authorities, particularly regarding the construction of poorhouses linked to the local churches. The basic approach remained unchanged – the local community was responsible for its own deserving poor, elderly and sick.[60]

The order of 1642 also gave detailed regulations for the poor and sick who would be cared for within the larger hospitals financed by the crown: the elderly and frail, who were unable to maintain themselves or had no relations to assist them; and the mentally ill and those who suffered from infectious diseases and had to be isolated from the rest of society. In this connection it is noteworthy that leprosy was spreading rapidly in Finland, Åland and eastern Sweden during the seventeenth century.[61]

Even in Finland attempts were made to implement the social control inherent in the order of 1642. Thus in 1654 the Count of Korsholma, Gabriel Bengtsson Oxenstierna, ordered the officials in his domains to arrest all male and female vagrants in accordance with the regulations of begging. They were to be sent to his estate of Korsholma and be put to work. Simultaneously the count ordered that servants and farm labourers needed to have their terms of employment fixed before Easter or Michaelmas day and to have arrived at their place of work within eight days of these dates if they wanted to avoid being arrested for vagrancy.[62]

Towards the end of the sixteenth century forced labour came to be seen as the only solution to vagrancy and begging by the undeserving poor. It was in this connection that a new poor relief institution was created in most major towns and cities in North-western Europe: the workhouse or house of correction. These institutions sought to combine social discipline and control with a general mercantilist economic policy which benefited society at large.[63] They gained a footing in Scandinavia during the first decades of the seventeenth century. The order of 1619, detailing the administration of market towns in Sweden, made it clear that all towns were expected to establish a combined workhouse and orphanage. But nothing happened until three years later, when Stockholm, as a result of the government decree concerning houses of correction and in accordance with developments in a number of major European cities, decided to establish a combined orphanage and workhouse where the inmates should treat and prepare cloth under the supervision of German clothiers. By 1625, however, only the clothworks supervised by immigrant craftsmen from northern Germany had come into existence. Six years later the institution came under the control of the admiral Clas Fleming, and after he became royal administrator of Stockholm in 1634, Fleming commenced the building of the orphanage which was finished in 1638. By the early 1640s the Stockholm authorities had begging children removed from the streets and incarcerated in this institution. But these children did not spend the whole day in the clothworks. They also attended school, where they were catechised in the main tenets of the Lutheran faith and taught to read and write. This limited education was not restricted to boys, as was often the case in early modern Europe, but also included girls. In spite of the emphasis on social control, it is noteworthy that the poor relief orders of 1642 and 1698 emphasised the importance of a proper Christian upbringing and education of poor and orphaned children.[64]

Generally, the children in the orphanage were between seven and fifteen years old. If we assume that the mortality rate was higher in Stockholm than in most other towns and cities of early modern Europe, then the mortality rate among the orphans was higher than the norm for the town and significantly higher than for their age group as such in Stockholm. These data are revealing about the conditions these children were exposed to. Thus it was not until the 1690s that the orphanage began to provide food for the children, who until then had relied on what they received from their employers, for whom they were forced to work.

Stockholm remained unique among the towns of seventeenth-century Sweden and Finland in having a combined workhouse and orphanage. Even if this institution had been created in order to help break the vicious circle of continuous begging and criminality within poor families, the authorities had primarily been motivated by economic, mercantilist considerations and the ambition to impose some form of social control on the growing number of destitute. This is clearly demonstrated by the close collaboration between the large clothworks on Södermalm, Barnäng, and the town's police during the 1670s. The police arrested children begging in the streets and sent them to Barnäng spinning mill, where they faced conditions much worse than their predecessors had encountered in the orphanage some decades earlier.[65]

Begging continued to represent a major problem for the authorities throughout the seventeenth century. A number of bills and solutions attempting to deal with the issue were drafted. The proposal of 1649–50 suggested a highly decentralised approach. Begging and all sorts of licences for beggars were to be prohibited. A regular poor rate was to be established which, had it been introduced, would have put considerable financial strain on the local parishes. Like a number of similar plans, it was rejected by the Estates, not least because of the economic implications.[66]

The goverment's inability to devise new and comprehensive schemes for poor relief and health care provision, which could generate the necessary support locally, constituted only part of the authorities' difficulties in this domain. The more limited statutes already introduced by the government were clearly not observed, but had repeatedly to be re-issued. For obvious reasons, the growing problem of poverty and begging proved acute in the capital, Stockholm, and a statute aimed at reinforcing and extending the 1642 poor relief order was issued in 1663. The most innovative element of this statute was the creation of a special body of poor-rate collectors – a semi-voluntary system which came close to a regular tax for the poor. Twice the government attempted to have this system extended to the whole country, but it was rejected by parliament in 1664 and again in 1668. These two bills constitute the last attempts of central government to reform an inadequate system of poor relief and health care provision in the seventeenth century. Thus the next major attempt of a comprehensive reform had to wait a century. Meanwhile the church order of 1686 and the poor relief order of 1698 only sought to enhance and enforce existing policies.[67]

The government's plan for a comprehensive reform in 1664 merits a closer look, not least because of its approach and attitude to the social problems of the day. It intended poor relief and health care to be centred in the major towns, and that each province should have a hospital, an orphanage and a house of correction or workhouse. These institutions were to be financed by a mixture of compulsory and voluntary contributions, the emphasis being on the former – only the amount was discretionary. Not surprisingly, the bill of 1664 continued to uphold the distinction between deserving and undeserving poor. Vagrants and idlers were to be prevented from begging and forced to work, and local authorities were warned not to be taken in by such people. Only those poor who had known better days and known some form of prosperity were treated charitably in this bill. Such former upright citizens were not to suffer the indignity of having to beg, but were to be looked after by special alms collectors and given special treatment in the provincial hospitals. This division of the deserving poor into a first and second class may well have been a reality from the third decade of the seventeenth century when the hospitals began to offer two forms of board – a cheaper option for the majority and the so-called *fogdespisordning* which cost three times more.[68]

A Finnish parallel to Rudbeckius's diocesan statutes can be found in the *Perbreves commonitiones* concerned with poor relief and health care, issued in 1673 by the active and learned Bishop of Åbo, Johannes Gezelius the elder. In accordance with the clergy's decision of 1672 he attempted to supplant begging with work for the able-bodied poor and alms from the local parishes. He instructed his clergy to restrict the number of begging licenses they issued, especially in connection with local fairs where begging was seen to contribute to the drunkenness and licentousness which prevailed at these occasions. He also warned his clergy against Gypsies and Lapps who roamed the countryside! Instead, in accordance with the Fathers, he recommended his flock to bring gifts for the poor when they attended service in their parish churches. They could then show their charitable inclination by giving such gifts to those poor who were waiting outside the church or in the porch before the start of the service.[69]

In his statutes Gezelius also demonstrated considerable concern for health care provision. Those suffering from infectious diseases were to be sent to the local hospital. The wealthy patients had to pay for their care while the local parishes were to pay for the poor. But an alternative was open to the wealthier citizens, who were allowed to remain at home if isolated in a separate building. The clergy were to pray for the infected not only privately, but publicly at Sunday services. During periods when an increasing number of sick people requested visits from their minister, the clergy were told not to visit the wealthiest and most influential members first, but those of their flock who were in greatest need.[70]

It was not until the church order of 1686 that responsibility for supervising the hospitals was expressly delegated to the royal district governor, the bishop, the local minister and the burgomaster. The district governor and the bishop were in charge, while day-to-day involvement rested with the minister and burgomaster. The 1686 order emphasised the obligation of the minister to visit and comfort even patients who suffered from infectious diseases. Larger towns were instructed to employ a special 'plague priest'.[71]

Swedish legislation of the early modern period, from the Stockholm statute of 1533 until the church order of 1686, demonstrates that little if anything had changed with regard to the clientele of the hospitals. By the end of the seventeenth century this still consisted of a mixture of poor, sick and elderly. The hospitals continued to operate as a combination of almshouses, nursing homes and medical institutions. The growing distinction between deserving and undeserving poor, and the authorities' attempt to exclude the latter group from public charity was undoubtedly a response to the strain on the system caused by the rapidly growing number of poor and destitute people who left the countryside to seek relief in the population centres. Neither indoor relief, in the form of parish infirmaries (where they had been established) and district hospitals, nor outdoor relief were able to provide the care and alms needed.[72]

Consequently the significance of begging grew as the only avenue of support open to the rapidly expanding number of destitute. Furthermore, the danger of being incarcerated in one of the new workhouses may well have made a fair number of the poor deeply suspicious of the indoor relief available and encouraged them to travel between farms, villages and towns.

Towards the end of the seventeenth century begging reached a plateau and started to decline, simultaneously taking on a more organised form. Thus at the summer court meeting at Lapua in Österbotten in 1681 it was announced that no non-local beggars were present in the parishes any longer. Two years later it can be seen from the local records of Södra Österbotten that so-called parish beggars were actively begging in accordance with the poor relief order of 1642. In spite of each community's obligation to care for its own poor, non-local beggars and vagrants continued to be a problem. Often when begging they behaved aggressively and threatened violence. Thus in 1691 the bishop of Åbo ordered that such scoundrels should be brought to court and punished.[73]

The shortage of qualified medical personnel in Sweden and Finland helps explain why proper medical institutions were slow in appearing. Two professors of medicine were employed at the University of Uppsala and one at the University of Åbo (founded in 1640) in the second half of the seventeenth century. The Åbo professor remained the only properly trained physician in Finland until the 1750s. But medical teaching remained old-fashioned and theoretical with little or no emphasis on clinical training. Until the mid-seventeenth century the only people to have experienced some practical medical training were the military barber-surgeons. The fact that in the second half of the seventeenth century a number of foreign barber-surgeons established themselves, first in Stockholm and then in remoter parts of the realm, is proof that public concern for, and awareness of medical provisions was growing. Vaasa in Österbotten could boast a barber-surgeon in 1648. In 1663 the post was occupied by the German Henrik Eggers, who used the title Surgeon. A surgeon may well have found it difficult to generate enough business for a decent income in this small, provincial Finnish town. Thus a decade later Eggers had changed his occupation to that of merchant. But by 1683 Vaasa had received its first publicly appointed district surgeon, who later passed his exams at the *Collegium Medicum* in Stockholm.[74]

The vast majority of the population continued to rely on popular healers and traditional herbal remedies throughout the seventeenth century. Cunning folk with their mixture of magic and traditional remedies offered the only available assistance in case of disease. But even with the few available physicians and surgeons, they could offer little or no help in the growing number of serious epidemics which ravaged Sweden and Finland in 1603, 1622 and 1657. As in the rest of Europe, the epidemics, mainly plague, spread from the major towns, the population centres, to the periphery. Thus those who attended the district court in Österbotten in Finland in 1657 were instructed to avoid any association with new arrivals from Sweden, where plague had broken out.

Leprosy caused similar reactions locally, but in spite of this not all lepers appear to have been incarcerated in infirmaries and hospitals. In 1654 the local court in Lapua in Österbotten decided that those peasants who did not transfer their wives who suffered from leprosy to the hospital were to have their houses demolished. Similarly, if anyone was found sheltering a leper, they were to pay a fine of forty silver marks. Nearly thirty years later, during the episcopal visitation of Isokyrö, the parishioners were admonished to send their lepers to hospital. At the same time the clergy was instructed to comfort the sick and infected, who were to receive the eucharist at the church porch or in the churchyard.[75]

Failed harvests at the beginning and end of the seventeenth century greatly affected Swedish and Finnish society. The crisis of the 1690s had an especially disastrous impact in Finland, and it has been estimated that about 100,000 Finns died of hunger or disease during this decade and the Finnish population shrank to 350,000. The health care and poor relief available proved totally inadequate in this situation, where permanent unemployment was already a serious problem. A massive population shift from the countryside to the urban centres resulted. Crowds of starved peasants sought assistance in the major towns of the realm; Stockholm in particular witnessed a massive influx. The government responded by ordering the establishment of rasp houses for men and spinning houses for women in all the major towns, naively expecting some solution to the social disruption by dealing firmly with those poor considered undeserving.[76]

As already mentioned, the intention of the church order of 1571 that most parishes should establish their own infirmaries or poor chambers had largely failed, even if the government continued to admonish local communities to act. As late as 1697 the crown once again admonished local communities to establish infirmaries, while simultaneously trying to encourage people to donate more money to the common chest or poor box, suggesting that collections should be made at family gatherings and local feasts.[77]

In 1699 the Bishop of Åbo, Johannes Gezelius the younger, suggested that parishioners should pay for the support of their own poor. A register of 'the destitute and very poor' should be drawn up and the local residents, according to their financial ability, should then pay for the support of those who had no relatives able to assist them. Thus Gezelius became instrumental in creating the rote system of relief, which from the start of the eighteenth century became the cornerstone of poor relief in Sweden and Finland. Traditionally the poor had collected their alms by following a fixed begging route which took them to certain local farms and houses at regular intervals, thus creating a voluntary system of relief. By the turn of the century it was transformed into the parish rote system whereby a certain number of local farms had undertaken to support one or more poor people who had been selected as so-called 'rote poor'. Undoubtedly this system constituted a marked improvement for those who were granted rote-poor status, and resulted in a vast improvement of public charity. But it never filtered through to the more distant and less populous regions of the realm, which still had to rely on traditional forms of voluntary relief throughout the eighteenth century.[78]

Local begging occasionally assumed peculiar forms in seventeenth century Sweden and Finland. In Stockholm special beggar corporations came into existence, among them one catering exclusively for Finnish beggars. Even if the legislation of the period attempted to exclude drifters and vagrants from relief, restricting it to the local poor, examples can be found of outsiders being permitted to beg. Thus in Kokkola in Österbotten in 1673 vagrants were allowed to remain in the town if they paid an annual fee to the authorities, either in cash or work. Generally, however, local authorities remained hostile to poor migrants, especially women, who were considered to offer unwanted competition to resident poor women, many of whom were active in unlicensed innkeeping and prostitution.[79] Town authorities often conducted raids to flush out non-resident poor, fining householders and landlords who sheltered them. In 1665 ten 'useless migrants' were expelled from Vaasa, while in Åbo those servants out of work had a choice between forced labour or work as carriers. The government's constant need for soldiers and sailors from the second half of the sixteenth century onwards constituted an even greater threat to the poor. Local authorities found that by conscripting vagrants and destitute members of their communities they solved two problems at once, finding the number of soldiers requested by central government while saving their communities unnecessary expenses on poor relief. That is, if they had not already found employment for such people in the newly established cloth works.[80]

From Olaus Petri's statutes of 1533 for the hospitals in Stockholm to the legislation for poor relief and health care provision of the late seventeenth century, there is a significant shift away from a primary concern for care of destitute and suffering members of the Protestant Christian community towards a concern for greater social control of the poor. This emphasis on control and stigmatisation of the poor, with its attempt to differentiate between the deserving and undeserving which eventually led to the creation of rasp-, spinning-, and workhouses, has been seen as the state's response to the growing problems of poverty and vagrancy. There is undoubtedly much evidence to support such an interpretation. Furthermore, the enthusiasm for care and Christian commitment evident in Olaus Petri's hospital statutes of 1533 would have been difficult to maintain for more than a generation, especially as the new, Protestant and locally accountable system of relief came under additional pressure from a society in flux. In this situation it was only natural for the growing government machinery to try to limit the available relief to the most deserving, while doing its utmost to prevent begging and vagrancy. But it should not be forgotten that simultaneously with this approach both local and central government did their best to protect the interest of the deserving poor. Stricter administrative controls of indoor as well as outdoor relief were repeatedly introduced in order to prevent abuse by those who administered it. It was, in other words, not only the poor who were exposed to greater control in this period. It remained a central aim for the authorities of post-Reformation Sweden and Finland to provide good Christian care and assistance based on neighbourly love, even if the definition of those who were considered deserving narrowed considerably over time as a consequence of the social and political climate of the day.

ACKNOWLEDGEMENTS

I thank Ole Peter Grell and Eljas Orrman for their expert advice and help with this chapter.

NOTES

1 Å. Sandholm, *Kyrkan och Hospitalshjonen. En undersökning rörande omsorgen om de sjuka och fattiga i välfärdsanstalterna i Finland*, Helsinki 1973, 11–12.
2 See B. Geremek, *Geschichte der Armut*, Munich/Zurich 1988, 43; see also W. Fischer, *Armut in der Geschichte. Erscheinungsformen und Lösungsversuche der 'Sozialen Frage' in Europa seit dem Mittelalter*, Göttingen 1982.
3 M. Morell, *Studier i den Svenska Livsmedelskonsumtionens Historia. Hospitalhjonens livsmedelskonsumtion 1621–1872*, Uppsala 1987, 77–80.

4   Sandholm, *Kyrkan och Hopitalshjonen*, 46–7; see also P. Pulma, 'Vaivaisten valtakunta', in J. Jaakkola *et al.* (eds) *Armeliaisuus, Yhteisöapu, Sosiaaliturva.* *Suomalaisen sosiaalisen turvan historia*, Helsinki 1994, 17.

5   Sandholm, *Kyrkan och Hospitalshjonen*, 472.

6   E. I. Kouri, 'The early Reformation in Sweden and Finland', in O. P. Grell (ed.) *The Scandinavian Reformation. From Evangelical Movement to Institutionalisation of Reform*, Cambridge 1995, 45.

7   K. Pirinen, *Suomen Kirkon Historia*, 1, Porvoo 1991, 375; Morrell, *Studier*, 81–2.

8   V. Granlund and J. A. Almquist (eds) *Konung Gustav den Förstes Registratur*, 8, Stockholm 1883, 289–97; C. Blom, *Tiggare, Tidstjuvar, Lättningar och Landstrykare. Studier av attityder och värderingar i skrån, stadgar, ordningar och lagförslag gällande den offentliga vården 1533–1664*, Lund 1992, 22–37.

9   Quoted in Blom, *Tiggare*, 23.

10 Morell, *Studier*, 82–4.

11 B. Lager-Kromnow, *Att vara Stockholmare på 1560-talet*, Uppsala 1992, 202–5; for Danviken Hospital, see also A. Klockhoff, *Danvikens Hospital. Dess rättsliga ställning*, 2 vols, Uppsala 1935.

12 This interpretation of the Stockholm statute of 1533 differs significantly from the most recent work in this field by Conny Blom, who appears to downplay the significance of the Reformation for changing the view and approach to disease and poverty in Sweden in this period. Compare Blom, *Tiggare*, 22–3 with 243–4. I am grateful to Ole Peter Grell for pointing this out to me.

13 Blom, *Tiggare*, 30, 243–58.

14 Pirinen, *Suomen Kirkon*, 375.

15 Sandholm, *Kyrkan och Hospitalshjonen*, 472.

16 Kouri, 'The early Reformations', 63.

17 Morell, *Studier*, 83.

18 See Lager-Kromnow, *Att vara Stockholmare*, 200, 208.

19 *ibid.*, 198–9.

20 See Pulma, 'Vaivaisten', 29.

21 F. Irsigler, 'Bettler und Dirnen in der städtischen Gesellschaft des 14.–16. Jahrhunderts', in T. Riis (ed.) *Aspects of Poverty in Early Modern Europe*, Odense 1986, 2, 180–5.

22 I owe this point to Ole Peter Grell. For Europe in general, see R. Jütte, 'Poor Relief and Social Discipline in Sixteenth-Century Europe', *European Studies*, 11, 1981, 25–52; see also R. Jütte, *Poverty and Deviance in Early Modern Europe*, Cambridge 1994, 198. For Sweden, see Morell, *Studier*, 85.

23 See Chapter 2 of this volume; and O. P. Grell, 'The Religious Duty of Care and the Social Need for Control', *Historical Journal*, 39, 1996, 257–63.

24 A. Winroth, *Om Tjänstehjonsförhållandet enligt Svensk Rätt*, 1, Uppsala 1878, 106.

25 E. Jutikkala, 'Labour Policy and the Urban Proletariat in Sweden and Finland during the Pre-Industrial Era', in Riis, (ed.) *Aspects of Poverty*,

2, 135–6. For the social strains generated by conscription, see N. E. Villstrand, *Anpassning eller Protest. Lokalsamhället inför utskrivningarna av fotfolk till den svenska krigsmakten 1620–79*, Åbo 1992.

26 J. Wilmi, *Isäntäväet ja palvelusväen pito 1600-luvulla ja 1700-luvun alkupuolella*, Jyväskylä 1991, 63–70; see also Pulma, 'Vaivaisten', 29.

27 K. Pirinen, *Savon historia*, 2, 1, Pieksämäki 1982, 160–97. For the parish of Kemi, see J. Koivisto, 'Pääpiirteitä Kemijokisuun Asutuskehityksestä', in M. Partanen (ed.) *Kotiseutuni Keminmaa*, Kemi 1988, 20–3. For the demographic developments, see also E. Jutikkala, *The Way Up. Desertion and land colonization in the Nordic countries c. 1300–1600*, Stockholm 1981, 120–38, 140–2; J. Myrdal, '1500-talets Bebyggelsesexpansion – en Forskningsöversikt', *Scandia* (1987), 77–98; J. Söderberg, 'Hade Heckscher rätt? Priser och reallöner i 1500-talets Stockholm', *Historisk Tidskrift* (Sweden), 1987, 349–55.

28 Blom, *Tiggare*, 57–64.

29 Lager-Kromnow, *Att Vara Stockholmare*, 200.

30 E. Färnström, *Om Källorna till 1571 Års Kyrkoordning Särskilt med Hänsyn till Tyska Kyrkoordningar*, Uppsala 1935; S. Kjöllerström, *Svenska Förarbeten till Kyrkoordningen av Är 1571*, Stockholm 1940; Kouri, 'The early Reformation', 64.

31 *Kyrkoordningar och Förslag dertill före 1686. Handlingar rörande Sveriges historia*, 2:2, Stockholm 1872, 175–80.

32 Pirinen, *Savon Historia*, 575–6.

33 Klockhoff, *Danvikens Hospital*, 1, 201–3; and Morell, *Studier*, 84–5.

34 See P. Slack, *Poverty and Policy in Tudor and Stuart England*, London 1988; and R. Jütte, *Poverty and Deviance*, 53–4. For Sweden, see J. Söderberg, 'La pauvreté en Suede 1500–1800', in T. Riis (ed.) *Aspects of Poverty in Early Modern Europe*, 3, Odense 1990, 106–29.

35 A. Stiernman (ed.) *Alla Riksdagars och Mötes Besluth samt Arfföreningar, Regementsformer, Försäkringar och Bewillningar*, 1, Stockholm 1728, 624–5.

36 Morell, *Studier*, 86.

37 E. Jutikkala, *Suomen Talonpojan Historia*, 2nd ed., Helsinki 1958, 208.

38 For the European poor laws and legislation in this period, see Slack, *Poverty and Policy* and Jütte, *Poverty and Deviance*.

39 For the order of 1624, see P. E. Thyselius (ed.) *Handlingar Rörande Svenska Kyrkans och Läroverkens Historia*, 1, Örebro 1839, 43–51. For the link between harvest failure, increase in incidence of disease and mortality, see for instance P. Slack, 'Mortality Crises and Epidemic Disease in England 1485–1610', in C. Webster (ed.) *Health, Medicine and Mortality in the Sixteenth Century*, Cambridge 1979, 10–59.

40 Blom, *Tiggare*, 100–1; for beggar kings, see Chapter 7 of this volume and L. Levander, *Fattigt Folk och Tiggare*, Stockholm 1934, 149–54.

41 Blom, *Tiggare*, 76–104. I owe this point to Ole Peter Grell.

42 B. Dahlberg, *Bidrag till Svenska Fattiglagstiftningens Historia*, Uppsala 1893, 47.

43 Morell, *Studier*, 88.

44 For leprosy in Scandinavia, see P. Richards, 'Leprosy in Scandinavia. A discussion of its origins, its survival, and its effect on Scandinavian life

over the course of nine centuries', *Medicinhistorisk Årbbok*, 1960, 113–25.

45   Morell, *Studier*, 89.

46   *Samling af Instructioner för Högre och Lägre Tjenstemän vid Landtregeringen i Sverige och Finland*, Stockholm 1852, 191–4.

47   Blom, *Tiggare*, 77, 83, 91.

48   E. I. Kouri, 'Statsmaktstänkandet i Början av nya Tiden', in E. I. Kouri, *Historiankirjoitus, Politiikka, Uskonto – Historiography, Politics, Religion*, Jyväskylä 1990, 270.

49   Ericus Erici, *Postilla*, 2, Stockholm 1625, 887–8.

50   E. I. Kouri, 'Der Einfluss der Deutschen Gebrauchsliteratur in Finnland im 17. Jahrhundert. Die Vorlagen von Ericus Ericis Postille', in Kouri, *Historiography*, 515–16. For Germany, see M. Stolleis, 'Grundzüge der Beamtenethik 1550–1650', *Verwaltung*, 13, 1980, 447–75.

51   M. Parvio, *Isaacus Rothovius. Turun piispa*, Helsinki 1959, 126–8.

52   H. Lundström (ed.) 'Johannes Rudbeckius' Kyrkio-stadgar för Westerås Stift', *Skrifter utg. av Kyrkohistoriska Förening*, 2, 1, Uppsala 1900, 52–62; for Finland, see A. Sandholm, *Klockarna i Finland på 1500- och 1600- Talen*, Åbo 1960, 33–6.

53   Sandholm, *Kyrkan och Hospitalshjonen*, 472–3.

54   Quoted in *ibid.*, 380–1.

55   Pulma, 'Vaivaisten', 23.

56   Quoted in Pulma, 'Vaivaisten', 34–5. For the elderly in particular, see M. Pelling, 'Old People and Poverty in Early Modern Towns', *The Society for the Social History of Medicine Bulletin*, 34, 1984, 42–7.

57   A. Luukko, *Etelä-Pohjanmaan Historia*, 3, Vaasa 1945, 776.

58   Sandholm, *Kyrkan och Hospitalshjonen*, 65–70; and Pulma, 'Vaivaisten', 31–3.

59   Luukko, *Etelä-Pohjanmaan*, 778–9; and P. Virrankoski, *Pohjois-Pohjanmaan ja Lapin Historia*, 3, Oulu 1973, 556.

60   A. A. von Stiernman (ed.) *Samling utaf Kongliga Bref/Stadgar och Förordningar*, 2, Stockholm 1750, 327–34; and Blom, *Tiggare*, 137–46.

61   Richards, 'Leprosy', 118–22.

62   Luukko, *Etelä-Pohjanmaan*, 778.

63   For Germany, see for instance H. Stekl, '"Labore et fame". Sozialdisziplinierung in Zucht- und Arbeits häusern des 17. und 18. Jahrhunderts', in C. Sachsse and F. Tennstedt (eds) *Soziale Sicherheit und Soziale Disziplinierung. Beiträge zu einer historischen Theorie der Sozialpolitik*, Frankfurt am Main 1986, 119–47; Jütte, *Poverty*, 169–77.

64   G. Utterström, *Fattig och Föräldralös i Stockholm på 1600- och 1700-Talen*, Umeå 1978, 174–5.

65   *ibid.*, 176.

66   Blom, *Tiggare*, 152–78.

67   *ibid.*, 192–218.

68   See above.

69 J. Gezelius, *Perbreves commonitiones eller Korta Påminnelser*, Åbo 1673; and P. Laasonen, *Johannes Gezelius Vanhempi*, Helsinki 1977, 257–9. For the authorities' fear of Gypsies in early modern Europe, see A. L. Beier, 'Vagrants and the Social Order in Elizabethan England', *Past and Present*, 64, 1974, 8; Slack, *Poverty and Policy*, 24, 96, 98, 104–5; and F. Egmond, *Underworlds. Organised crime in the Netherlands 1650–1800*, Oxford 1993, 87–105. For vagrancy, see A. L. Beier, *Masterless Men. The vagrancy problem in England 1560–1640*, London 1985.

70 Laasonen, *Gezelius*, 255, 259.

71 Sandholm, *Kyrkan och Hospitalshjonen*, 386.

72 Morell, *Studier*, 88.

73 Luukko, *Etelä-Pohjanmaan*, 778 and P. Lempiäinen, *Piispan- ja Rovastintarkastukset Suomessa ennen Isoavihaa*, Helsinki 1967, 210.

74 M. Klinge, *Eine Nordische Universität. Die Universität Helsinki 1640–1990*, Helsinki 1992, 118; for Vaasa, see Luukko, *Etelä-Pohjanmaan*, 778.

75 Luukko, *Etelä-Pohjanmaan*, 780, 783. See also C. Johansen, 'Faith, Superstition and Witchcraft in Reformation Scandinavia' in O. P. Grell (ed.) *The Scandinavian Reformation*, 194, 203. For an excellent example of the effects of plague on an early modern society, see P. Slack, *The Impact of Plague in Tudor and Stuart England*, London 1985.

76 E. Jutikkala, 'The Great Finnish Famine in 1696–7', *Scandinavian Economic History Review*, 3, 1955, 50–55. For the population of Finland, see S. Koskinen *et al.* (eds) *Suomen väestö*, Helsinki 1994, 37–8.

77 P. Laasonen, *Suomen Kirkon Historia*, 3, Porvoo 1991, 241.

78 Sandholm, *Kyrkan och Hospitalshjonen*, 31–3.

79 For the connection between vagrancy, poverty, prostitution and alehouses, see P. Clark, *The English Alehouse. A social history 1200–1830*, London 1983, 110–12. For prostitution, see P. Schuster, *Das Frauenhaus. Städische Bordelle in Deutschland 1350 bis 1600*, Paderborn 1992; and O. Hufton, *The Prospect Before Her. A history of women in Western Europe*, 1 (1500–1800), London 1995.

80 Pulma, 'Vaivaisten', 30.

Chapter 9

Health care and poor relief in Danzig (Gdansk)

The sixteenth- and first half of the seventeenth century

Maria Bogucka

GENERAL REMARKS

Danzig in the early modern era was a prosperous Baltic port of 30–40,000 inhabitants in the sixteenth century and about 100,000 in the first half of the seventeenth century.[1] In the social structures of Danzig the proportion of poor people – that is of those who were not paying any urban taxes – could be estimated at the beginning of the sixteenth century at between 20 and 25 per cent of the total population and was rising constantly.[2]

The town had a diversified commercial and industrial economy and was built around the greatest port of the Baltic region.[3] Since Danzig was bursting with trade and offered excellent opportunities for different jobs it was a focus of a constant stream of immigrants – permanent as well as temporary. Seamen, foreign merchants, craftsmen, wandering journeymen, Polish noblemen and their servants, poor people of both sexes seeking support through begging or temporary work – all these people were daily coming to the city. Some of them had no money to pay for their food and shelter, others who came for a short stay had to prolong their sojourn because of sudden illness. Such transients who lacked family or friends to look after them were a serious problem in most port cities. Thus illness and poverty were important social phenomena that met with a social response from municipal authorities as well as from individual town dwellers.

POOR RELIEF

The victory of the Reformation and the new approach to the problem of poverty resulted in Danzig in changes to poor relief organisation.[4] An urban law passed in 1525 stated that beggars should be mustered. All people able to work must leave the town; those coming back would be punished by marking one ear; if caught a second time they were to be imprisoned and sentenced to work in jail for life. Only the very ill and the weak were to be offered lodging in the town's hospitals, but even in these institutions they were to perform some work according to their abilities.[5] The innkeepers were warned not to shelter any beggars or 'idle people' and all parents were admonished not to allow their children to speak to or even approach a beggar.[6]

A second poverty law was passed in 1551. The city was divided into districts headed by special beggars' officers. They had to muster all beggars periodically; foreign ones were to be expelled from the city; local beggars genuinely in need of help were to be registered and given tokens allowing them to beg alms in strictly determined places.[7] In spite of these laws, similar to those issued across the whole of Europe in this period,[8] the city was full of beggars of both sexes, and rich burghers complained that they were constantly molested by poor people, often sick or invalid, both men and women, old people as well as children, who begged for money or bread.[9] Some of these poor were even dying on the streets.[10] The problem was very acute because of the association of beggars with criminality; indeed, many thefts were committed by beggars. They also acted as snoopers and feelers, gathering information for robbers and organised gangs; female beggars were often suspected of prostitution or even of witchcraft, and were feared because of their 'evil eye'.

To control this poverty the town authorities tried to develop and improve the network of urban hospitals. Since the Middle Ages there had been several hospitals in Danzig:

- In the city centre: the Hospital of the Holy Spirit (established 1253, extended in the sixteenth century by developing the so-called Back Hospital), as well as the Hospital of St Elisabeth (established before 1308) and the Hospital of St Jacob (established in 1414).
- In the suburbs: the Hospital of St Barbara (established in 1378), the Hospital of St Gertrud (established in 1342), the Smallpox Hospital with the so-called Lazaretto (end of the fifteenth Century, extended in 1542 by a Hospital for Mental Illness), the Hospital of Corpus Christi (established before 1385), the Hospital of All God's Angels (1380), and the Pestilence Hospital (1454).[11]

Altogether there were nine urban hospitals, each richly endowed with land and annuities. For instance St Jacob's Hospital owned large meadows at the outskirts of the city and several parcels of land in the city.[12] The Hospital of the Holy Spirit owned six villages, the St Elisabeth Hospital five to seven villages.[13] Besides plots of land in the countryside and parcels of land in the city, hospitals owned annuities and collected rents allotted to them in foundations and legacies made by town authorities, guild brotherhoods and individual rich burghers.[14] They also used casual alms collected by the hospital officers, sometimes by hospital lodgers themselves. In the middle of the sixteenth century a special institution called a Charity Board (*Spendeamt*) was established to seek alms and distribute the sums collected among individual beggars as well as among the hospitals.[15]

Hospitals, as can be seen from their accounts, had large sums of money at their disposal – thousands of Prussian Marks yearly.[16] No wonder that the office of hospital supervisor was regarded with envy as a very profitable business; that many conflicts occurred over who controlled hospitals; and accusations of fraud in hospital accounts were made throughout the sixteenth century.[17] As early as 1546, stricter control by the town council over hospitals was demanded and established.[18] At the beginning of the seventeenth century a new attempt was made to improve poor relief: in 1606 the financial arrangements as well as the administration of five main hospitals (St Elisabeth, the Holy Spirit, the Back Hospital, the Smallpox Hospital, and the Pestilence Hospital) were united and put under the closer supervision of the Charity Board. In 1610 the Board was given a new constitution which gave it better control over all the hospitals as well as over all the city's poor.[19]

In spite of the reform, the hospitals retained their twofold character as both poorhouses for old and invalid people, and simultaneously as infirmaries for the temporarily sick. The majority of Danzig's hospitals, however, were hospices, for instance St Jacob's Hospital (where old and crippled seamen were lodged),[20] or the Hospital of the Holy Spirit, the St Gertrud Hospital, the St Elisabeth, as well as the Corpus Christi Hospital. Only the Pestilence Hospital and the Smallpox Hospital with its Lazaretto had the character of infirmaries.

Although numerous, the hospitals were inadequate to the needs of a quickly expanding city. In spite of the fact that hospitals were rebuilt and extended during the sixteenth century, each of them could accommodate only a few people. St Jacob's Hospital, for instance, could keep only thirteen poor sailors, together with a number of wealthier seamen who could pay for their stay in the institution. Altogether in this hospital were lodged probably between twenty and thirty people.[21] In the year 1545 in the Hospital of St Elisabeth there were forty-five people accommodated, while in the Holy Spirit there were twenty-eight.[22] It is estimated that altogether Danzig's hospitals could house probably 300–400 people. This was very few considering the needs of the several thousand resident poor.

There was great competition for getting a place in the hospitals and it was certainly not the poorest individuals who were always the winners. In the sixteenth- and seventeenth centuries the most popular form of introduction into a hospital was by the purchase of residence, an opportunity which arose only on the death of a previous lodger. Between the end of the sixteenth century and the beginning of the seventeenth (before the great devaluation of the Prussian Mark in 1619–21) the price varied between twenty and 200 Prussian Marks.[23] These were rather substantial prices. The big difference in them could serve as evidence of a significant material differentiation among the hospitals' lodgers. Often they were not really poor people and their probate inventories confirm such suspicions. Among the hospitals' lodgers there were people who owned some money which they used to lend to people in need; besides cash and loan bills, inventories often list respectable people's belongings, for instance good garments or even pieces of jewellery. On 12 February 1641, the Hospital of Corpus Christi sold the belongings of two of its dead lodgers for the not inconsiderable sum of fifty-seven Prussian Marks.[24] At the beginning of the year 1612 the same hospital received 100 Prussian Marks due from debtors of one of its lodgers.[25] In the year 1619 the Hospital of Corpus Christi sold belongings of its dead lodgers for fifty-two Prussian Marks and received 800 Prussian Marks as returned loans.[26]

The probate inventories of two women who died in the Pestilence Hospital have been preserved. The wife of Hans Kuren, who died on 12 December 1608, left some garments (four shirts, two bonnets, one towel, one napkin, five collars, one cap, one fur coat, one blue dress of coarse cloth, one old coat), one brass cauldron, one tripod, one shelf, one barrel, one pail and a few bedclothes (one featherbed, one sheet – the second one 'she took with her to the grave' – one pillow and one mattress). She left some debts to be paid, together totalling fifty-eight Prussian Marks. Her funeral cost forty-eight Prussian Marks and six Pennies.[27] Before she was accepted into the hospital she had been ill at home for three months.

On 30 August 1609 a woman called Elisabeth (the last name is not mentioned) died in the same hospital. She left some modest garments and bedclothes as well as a small 'treasury' – a silver scale and silver belt both pawned for twenty Prussian Marks (the cash, however, was not found). She also owned five books, three painted glass vases, thirteen paintings, one 'painted letter to hang on the wall', one painting on wood and five small pictures printed on paper (woodcuts?). Her funeral cost fifty-three Prussian Marks.[28]

Both lists show some degree of wealth, in the second case the existence of objects associated with culture and education (books!). Both of the cited inventories are, however, not typical of our theme: they present the belongings not of a permanent hospital lodger, but only of a temporary one.

The conditions of life in a hospital were very much differentiated. They depended mostly on the route of admission to the hospital: the poor accepted without any fee had to be satisfied with modest conditions, while people who had bought their residence were offered some privileges. There were basic rooms where two or more people had to share one bed, but some lodgers were given their own bed or even their own private room.[29] The duty to work (cleaning, wood cutting, water carrying, helping in the kitchen) was also shared unequally. The same was the case with personal discipline (limited rights to invite guests, a prohibition on leaving the hospital premises without permission, prohibition on returning late at night, etc.). Each offence was punished by different penalties: reprimand, food deprivation or even expulsion from the institution.

All lodgers, without regard to their wealth and status in the hospital, were united in prayers and large religious ceremonies, which took up a great part of the daily routine in each hospital. Prohibitions on fighting, stealing, name-calling and abusing fellow inmates, which are included in all hospital ordinances, testify that life within the institution was not always harmonious.[30]

Meals were also differentiated, depending on the status of lodgers, despite the fact that food was mainly served in a common room. Hospital accounts list large sums spent on purchasing meat, fish, butter, peas and groats; farms owned by the hospitals produced milk and cheese, fruit and vegetables.[31] For drink, cheap beer was served.[32] It seems that food in the hospitals was varied and perhaps much better than that available to individual poor living on their own. At the end of the sixteenth- and on the threshold of the seventeenth century, in Corpus Christi Hospital on average 760 Prussian Marks were spent on food yearly.[33] Assuming that the hospital sheltered thirty-five people this would give twenty-two Prussian Marks per person, that is one penny daily, the same as a hard working journeyman received towards his food.[34] It means that food in hospitals was not scarce. The problem, however, was its distribution; probably the largest share went to the hospital officers and wealthy lodgers, while the poor had to be satisfied with leftovers. Hence the complaints from one side and the ban on rejecting food on the other, as well as the prohibitions on food stealing or taking food out and selling it outside the hospital.[35]

In cold seasons the hospitals were heated – the accounts usually list the expenses for firewood. Expenses for musicians and singers are also mentioned, probably connected with the religious ceremonies performed in these institutions.[36]

Hospitals were not the only institutions dedicated to poor relief. In the year 1542 a Home for Children was established close to St Elisabeth's Hospital; at first both establishments had a common administration and finances. The Home for Children was meant to solve one of the important problems of the quickly expanding maritime town: the care of numerous illegitimate children, of foundlings and orphans. The institution could, however, foster at most forty children, which seriously limited its role. In 1552, King Sigismund Augustus issued a special privilege giving to the charity boys and girls the same rights which the children of legal birth enjoyed.[37] The Home was directed by four supervisors appointed by the town council. Here also a fee for admission was required and sometimes a substantial one: from ten to 2,000 Polish Florins! We do not know the proportion of poor to more wealthy children accepted into the Home, but competition for admission was probably great. The majority of admitted children were infants (hence the several wet nurses on the staff), but older ones may also have been accepted. The nurslings were kept in the Home till their adolescence. They were taught to read, write and do some arithmetic as well as to perform some practical manual jobs; above all, however, they learned to pray and to sing religious songs and psalms.[38] We know very little about the conditions of life in the Home, but from casual evidence they were probably quite tolerable. Food and garments were largely provided by donations made by rich merchants.

Rising criminality, especially youth delinquency, resulted in 1629 in the establishment of a workhouse.[39] Here the men, women and children had to learn social discipline by hard work, prayers and hunger; all offences, even minor transgressions, were to be punished by confiscation of meals and floggings. It was a classical kind of workhouse, organised on the Dutch pattern (after the model of Amsterdam's workhouse), with men rasping Brazilian wood or weaving cloth, women spinning, and children combing wool. The working hours in summer were from four to nine o'clock, in winter from five to nine, and the food ration was extremely small. Only very efficient workers received some extra pay with which they were allowed to buy extra food.[40]

As we can see from this short survey, poor relief in Danzig encompassed several kinds of institutions: hospitals for adults, an orphanage and a workhouse. The purpose of all these institutions was not only to ease the life of the poor, but also to control them, and to limit the danger of poverty disturbing social stability or resulting in criminality. But in spite of considerable resources accorded to it, poor relief and the network of charity establishments were too weak to solve the problems of the rapidly increasing numbers who were in need of help. Admission to hospitals as well as to the orphanage constituted a field of bitter competition which resulted in the favouring of the upper strata of poverty; the very poor, those without any financial resources, had little chance of becoming hospital lodgers. Hence the great number of beggars in Danzig and the constant increase in numbers of the socially marginal, including thieves and prostitutes.

The inadequacy of institutional poor relief resulted in the survival of individual charity in spite of the new attitudes toward poverty introduced by the Reformation. Beggars, often invalid or sick, were visible in the streets, lying in front of churches and other buildings, seeking shelter within town gates or in the hollows in town walls. In cold weather it was not rare to find a dead person on the street. In spite of the Reformation's rejection of good works as expressed in charitable giving, rich merchants still eased their conscience by giving alms and donating large sums to poor people in their wills. In the year 1564 Conrad and Barbara von Suchten offered the city the capital of 15,000 Prussian Marks for a yearly rent of 1,000 Marks, from which 100 Marks were to be distributed among the poor, 100 Marks given to the orphans and 100 Marks to the Smallpox Hospital. Other wills were less generous, but amounts from 1,000 to 1,500 Marks were often bequeathed to the poor, as well as garments and food. For instance in the second half of the sixteenth century a rich merchant, Anthony Ulrich, offered 1,500 Marks

> davon 60 Mrk Zinsen alle Jahr fallen, wofur man den elenden Kindern des Waisenhauses und den anderen personen auf den Tag Ulrici eine Mahlzeit anrichten soll: nemlich eine Tonne Bier, einen halben Ochsen, item Grutz mit Milch gekocht und einen Jedem einen Strutzel von 2 Groschen.[41]

Beggars and poor people were invited to funerals, and for their attendance and prayers were given food as well as small sums of money. All these donations were, however, insufficient and the expanding town had to cope with a growing margin of poverty and social discontent.

HEALTH CARE

As mentioned above, hospitals were above all poorhouses and not medical institutions. But they did supply certain medical services. The Smallpox Hospital had a medical doctor and a barber-surgeon among its personnel who attended sick people admitted to this institution. The Pestilence Hospital and Lazaretto were also institutions with medical functions. In other hospitals physicians and barbers were called in as required; in cases of need some medicines were distributed among the lodgers without charge.

As a large maritime city, Danzig had to cope with several diseases. The town's area of little more than 200 hectares was literally crammed with people. Sanitation facilities were inadequate. Only few rich houses had their own water supply, special bathrooms and well arranged privies. The level of personal hygiene was low. Most people lived close together: five or six to a room, sleeping two or three to a bed, sharing towels, eating from one bowl. As a result, contagious diseases were easily spread either by direct contact between individuals via the respiratory system, or by use of the same utensils, or transferred by insects such as fleas and lice. Venereal diseases spread rapidly mainly because of the influx to Danzig of large numbers of single men. The coastal climate of the city – cold and damp – as well as the insufficient heating and the use of cellars for housing the poor, resulted in a high frequency of rheumatic and pulmonary ailments. Dirt in kitchens, as well as stale food, must have caused a number of digestive troubles.

The frequency of bodily injuries resulted from the rough conditions of daily life as well as from the conditions of work on shipboard, at the harbour or in the workshops. Hard work, performed without suitable protection, caused numerous accidents. The typical diet of the poor inhabitants of Danzig was composed mostly of grain, and, lacking in vitamins and protein, resulted in anaemia, scurvy and a generally low individual resistance to contagious diseases. Over-nutrition – too much meat, animal fat, alcohol – caused heart and circulatory troubles among the wealthy burghers.[42]

Illness in the early modern period was primarily a family affair. The bedridden were attended by other family members, mostly women. But not everyone in Danzig had family around their sickbed. The number of single people in this large maritime city was growing throughout the period under consideration.[43] An even more complicated problem was posed by the influx of people coming to the city for a short stay, usually for some weeks only. Such visitors were especially numerous in summer, when the harbour was busy.

Since the Middle Ages guilds and journeymen brotherhoods had organised special 'sickrooms' in their inns, where ill wandering craftsmen (also local ones, but only those without family or their masters' support) could find bed and care.[44] In the sixteenth- and seventeenth centuries such sickrooms and dispensaries were organised by furriers, tawers, cartwrights, wheelwrights, coopers, pailmakers, carpenters, pewterers, nailmakers, gunsmiths, cutlers, blacksmiths, coppersmiths, butchers, ship carpenters, bricklayers, saddlers, beltmakers and potters.[45] At the beginning of the seventeenth century, carpenters tried to establish a sickroom for their journeymen in one of the municipal hospitals.[46] To take care of a sick person in such a room, a woman was usually hired, and sometimes other journeymen also gave their services to help sick colleagues.[47] The problem of taking care of sick journeymen was so important that it was the main reason why masters and town authorities allowed several journeymen's brotherhoods to be established in Danzig.[48]

But the journeymen's sickrooms and dispensaries solved the needs of one social group only. Danzig's influx of sailors and foreign merchants as well as people from the Polish hinterland (noblemen as well as their servants and craftsmen) resulted in complications if they were suddenly taken ill. The hospital of St Jacob was dedicated, as mentioned above, to the permanent care of old sailors, and could not offer any help to those seamen who came to Danzig for a short stay and fell ill.[49] St Barbara's Hospital in the suburbs should theoretically have taken care of Polish raftsmen,[50] but as a hospice it could not afford to admit the sick for a short stay and cure. The growing need to help sick visitors to the city resulted in the emergence of a network of inns providing them with a bed, meals appropriate to contemporary ideas of good diet (white bread, wine, nourishing soups) and the care of a doctor or a barber as well as of nursing women.[51] The level of services depended on a patient's means; in the event of death the innkeeper usually arranged the funeral, covering his expenses by selling the belongings of the departed.[52]

THE MENTAL AND MEDICAL RESPONSE TO ILLNESS

There were two characteristic responses to illness in early modern Danzig: one resulting from the pervasiveness of the Protestant faith on citizens' mentality, and the second resulting from the lively contacts between 'learned' and 'popular' culture. Both attitudes were fused into one system of beliefs which enabled individuals to cope with the terrifying phenomena of illness and death.

As faithful adherents of the Lutheran or Calvinist creed, the inhabitants of Danzig saw illness as God's punishment for their sins, and at the same time as an antechamber to death, the gateway leading to a better existence.[53] Their striving for a stoic response to suffering was linked to the idea of predestination, popular in Danzig not only among Calvinists. Pain was regarded as the inevitable path to redemption and eternity. It was, however, logical to conclude that an illness inflicted by God could not be cured without God's help and consent. Medical treatment was therefore accompanied by prayers, and some physicians were bold enough to claim that God was their special ally.[54]

Religious attitudes to illness were confirmed by some 'learned' theories in which health and illness were regarded as phenomena subordinated to astral influences. Renaissance medicine had fortified the traditional belief in the unity of nature, a unity that encompassed God and the stars at one extreme and humanity and the terrestrial world at the other; it therefore seemed reasonable to assume that the stars would influence human life and especially human health. In sixteenth- and seventeenth-century Danzig, many scholars and physicians, such as Bartholomew Wagner, Severin Goebel and Willem Misocacus, agreed that astral influences moulded the state of a person's physical condition. Such attitudes led inevitably to natural magic, which spread among the educated inhabitants of Danzig in the form of several 'learned' theories, as well as among other citizens as witchcraft practices pretending to cure every ailment. The gap between 'learned' and 'popular' issues was not very wide.

Danzig in the sixteenth- and seventeenth centuries was an important centre of medical knowledge.[55] The High School established in the town in the middle of the sixteenth century was of university standard; in the first half of the seventeenth century it obtained the title of Academic School. Danzig maintained lively relations with the best European universities. A great influence on medicine in Danzig had been the famous John Placetomus, who in the second half of the sixteenth century introduced new ideas about the functioning of the human body. The leading physicians in Danzig were Christopher Heyll, who translated and commented on the works of Galen, and Adrian Pauli who worked on problems of diet and personal hygiene. Knowledge of anatomy was advancing rapidly; the first public dissection of a human corpse in Danzig was performed in 1613 by Joachim Oelhaf.[56] In 1643 his son Dr Nicholas Oelhaf published a herbal enumerating 350 plants from the Danzig region and describing their medicinal properties. Laurentius Eichstadt, a professor of anatomy in the years 1645–60, author of an eminent book on osteology and an expert on blood circulation, also achieved some fame. In the 1660s another physician, John Schmidt, tried intravenous injection of medicine on his patients; and some modern theories of blood circulation were developed by Dr Israel Conradt.

How big was the gap between this learned pinnacle of the medical world and average medical practice in Danzig? At the beginning of the seventeenth century the daily treatment of patients was still based primarily on the ideas of the ancients Hippocrates and Galen. Structurally the medical community of Danzig was composed of five distinct layers:

1 physicians or *promoti doctores*, trained in foreign universities and well experienced;

2 mostly self-taught surgeons;
3 barber-surgeons;
4 apothecaries;
5 unlicensed or non-professional healers of all kinds.[57]

At the top was the highly trained elite, the physicians – limited by the municipal authorities to between ten and twenty in number. In about 1530 the post of chief doctor or 'town physician' was created; his duty was to supervise the medical activities conducted by his colleagues. Surgeons and apothecaries had to prove their skill before him in order to obtain a license. In 1636 a collective supervisory body was established: the *Collegium Medicum*. It was a kind of Chamber of Medicine with the power to control medical affairs in the city. Anyone who wanted to get into medical practice in Danzig was obliged to present himself and his diploma before the *Collegium* and to pass an examination; in 1677 the duty to deliver a public lecture was added to the requirements.

Regulations improved the level of medical services. Blood letting and purgations were still in popular use, but there were also attempts to make individual diagnoses. Patients were carefully examined, their urine tested, their pulse and temperature checked. Physicians used both dietary prescriptions as well as chemical or herbal remedies. The dense network of dispensaries offered easy access to a wide range of syrups, powders, ointments and pills. Danzig had two town apothecary shops, one in the Main Town and another in the Old Town, which were put out on lease to some learned people. In addition there were many small private establishments, controlled by the town's physicians.[58]

Alongside learned medicine, popular healing continued to be widely practised. It was based on traditional folklore as well as on belief in magic amulets, secret miraculous remedies and witchcraft. Such beliefs were also shared by members of enlightened circles, who often resorted to the help of unofficial healers. Quacks were numerous in spite of fierce protests from learned professionals.

Women played a considerable role in popular medicine. The task of attending the sick was traditionally a female duty which over the centuries had enabled women to acquire a substantial body of medical knowledge. Women attended not only members of their own families but also ailing neighbours or foreign visitors in need. Women traditionally held a monopoly on delivering babies. Only in the richest families had calling a doctor to childbed come into practice in the seventeenth century; middle-class women were attended by a professional midwife.[59] In 1610 Danzig had established an official post of 'town midwife' with an annual salary of 100 marks, to attend women of wealthier families as well as to supervise the activities of other professional midwives. She was also obliged to testify in the court of justice in cases where infanticide was suspected.[60]

Analysis of Danzig's records shows that the incidence of professional medical care by physicians and barbers was rising in the town, especially in the seventeenth century.[61] The sources also show that acute illness in the seventeenth century was usually of short duration in Danzig: of 162 cases studied, 105 (64 per cent) resulted in death within one week, twenty-nine (18 per cent) within one month, twenty (12 per cent) within two months; in seven cases (4 per cent) the illness lasted more than one year.[62]

One might assume that the lack of more sophisticated treatment did not allow sick people in a critical condition to stay alive longer than a few days or weeks. But another explanation is also possible: the records analysed mostly concern the poor, and these probably only sought professional help *in extremis*, in order to avoid the high cost of treatment for as long as possible. Unfortunately we do not possess any statistics concerning the duration of illness among the wealthier inhabitants of Danzig.

Because of the limited dimensions of this study it is not possible to include an assessment of the epidemics, which plagued sixteenth- and seventeenth-century Danzig with extraordinary frequency and high mortality. This needs to be investigated separately.

CONCLUSIONS

1 In spite of extensive provisions, poor relief in Danzig in the sixteenth- and first half of the seventeenth century did not meet the great needs of the expanding maritime city. It resulted in the survival of traditional forms of charity (individual alms-giving, the poor begging on the streets) along with the development of institutional forms such as hospitals, an orphanage and a workhouse.

2 Health care outside the family was organised in the form of several institutions: hospitals, guild dispensaries, private sickrooms. The existence of such establishments was important in a large port

where many visitors fell ill without family or friends to attend them.

3 Along with the learned, rather well developed medicine, popular healing, consisting of extensive use of traditional remedies including some witchcraft practices, also existed in Danzig. The gap between learned and popular medicine was narrow. Both regarded illness as a punishment inflicted by God which could not be cured without God's help. Pain should be met with patience and stoicism. But in spite of the popularity of such ideas, the inhabitants of Danzig were eager to try every wonder medicine that promised to cure them.

NOTES

1 Maria Bogucka, 'Danzig and der Wende zur Neuzeit: von der Aktivon Handelsstadt zum Stapel und Produktionszentrum', *Hansische Geschichtsblätter*, 102 Jg., 1984, 95.

2 *Historia Gdanska* (*History of Danzig*), ed. Edmund Cieslak, vol. II, Danzig 1982, 552.

3 Maria Bogucka, 'Amsterdam and the Baltic in the First Half of the Seventeenth Century', *Economic History Review*, second series, XXVI, no. 3, 1973, 433–47.

4 Maria Bogucka, 'Przemiany Form Zycia w Gdansku u Progu Ery Nowo Zytnej' ('Changes in the Forms of Life in Danzig at the Threshold of Early Modern Times'), *Kwartalnik Historyczny* no. 4, 1982, 547 ff.; Zdzislaw Kropidlowski, *Formy Opieki nad Ubogimi w Gdansku od XVI do XVIII w.* (*Poor Relief in Danzig in the Sixteenth- to Eighteenth Centuries*), Danzig 1992, *passim*.

5 Paul Simson, *Geschichte der Stadt Danzig*, vol. II, Danzig 1918, 77.

6 *ibid.*

7 *ibid.*

8 See Wolfram Fischer, *Stadtische Armut und Armenfürsorge im 15 und 16. Jh.*, Göttingen 1979, *passim*.

9 Bogucka, 'Przemiany', 548.

10 *ibid.*

11 See Reinhold Curicke, *Der Stadt Danzig Historische Beschreibung*, Amsterdam-Danzig 1689, 342 ff.

12 Maria Bogucka, *Gdanscy Ludzie Morza w XVI–XVIII w.* (*Seamen in Danzig in the Sixteenth- to Eighteenth Centuries*), Danzig 1984, 101 ff.

13 Kropidlowski, *Formy Opieki*, 76 ff. Danzig Archives (hereafter AG) 300, 61/96; 300, R/Rr q 5.

14 Kropidlowski, *Formy Opieki*, 38 ff.

15 *ibid.*

16 See the accounts of the Holy Spirit and the St Elisabeth Hospitals for the years 1587–99, AG 300, R/Rr q 5; as well as Corpus Christi Hospital for the years 1609–19, AG 300, 61/96, 98, 104.

17 Kropidlowski, *Formy Opieki*, 48 ff.; Bogucka, *Gdanscy Ludzie Morza*, 103.
18 Simson, *Geschichte*, 187, 191, 390, 543.
19 Kropidlowski, *Formy Opieki*, 45 ff.
20 Bogucka, *Gdanscy Ludzie Morza*, 101–5.
21 Bogucka, *Gdanscy Ludzie Morza* 105.
22 Kropidlowski, *Formy Opieki*, 81.
23 AG 300, R/Rr q 5, 300, 61/96–104.
24 AG 300, 61/97.
25 AG 300, 61/98.
26 AG 300, 61/104.
27 AG 300, R/Vv 117, 232–23. Her husband was ill for six months, but had not died, *ibid.*
28 AG 300, R/Vv 117, 274–5.
29 Kropidlowski, *Formy Opieki*, 106. See also Ag 300, 61/104.
30 Bogucka, *Gdanscy Ludzie Morza*, 102; Kropidlowski, *Formy Opieki*, 103 ff. See also Chapter 8 of this volume.
31 Their own food was largely produced by, for instance, the St Jacobs, St Elisabeth and Holy Spirit Hospitals; see Maria Bogucka, *Organizacja Szpitalnictwa w Gdansku w XVI–XVII w. (Organisation of Hospitals in Danzig in the Sixteenth- to Seventeenth Centuries)*, forthcoming.
32 *ibid.*
33 AG 300, 61/96–104.
34 *Historia Gdanska*, 554; Maria Bogucka, *Gdańsk Jako Osrodek Produkcyjny od XIV do XVII w (Danzig as Production Centre from the Fifteenth to the Seventeenth Century)*, Warsaw 1962, 332 ff.
35 Kropidlowski, *Formy Opieki*, 104 ff.
36 *ibid.*, 94, 106.
37 *ibid.*, 116.
38 *ibid.*, 116.
39 Maria Bogucka, 'Les Origines de la Pensée Penitentiaire Moderne en Pologne du 17e s.', *Acta Poloniae Historica*, vol. 56, 1987, 19–28.
40 *ibid.*
41 Gottfried Loschin, *Beitraege zur Geschichte Danzigs und seiner Umgebung*, vol. II, Danzig 1837, 67.
42 Maria Bogucka, 'Illness and Death in a Maritime City: the case of Danzig in the seventeenth century', *The American Neptune*, vol. 51, no. 2, Spring 1991, 91–104.
43 Bogucka, 'Illness', 97.
44 Bogucka, *Gdansk Jako Osrodek Produkcyjny*, 352.
45 *ibid.*
46 AG 300, C/ 1766, 1770, 1772.
47 Bogucka, *Gdansk Jako Osrodek Produkcyjny*, 352.
48 *ibid.*
49 Bogucka, *Gdanscy Ludzie morza*, 103 ff.
50 Kropidlowski, *Formy Opieki*, 78.
51 Bogucka, *Gdanscy Ludzie Morza*, 103 ff.; *idem*, 'Illness', 97 ff.; *idem*, 'Smierc Niezamoznego Mieszkanca Miasta u Progu Ery Nowozytnej' ('Death of a Poor Towndweller on the Threshold of Modern Times'),

in Andrzej Wyrobisz and Michal Tymowski wiekach, eds, *Gzas-przestrzen-praca w dawnych wiekach,* Warsaw 1991, 285–9.

52 Bogucka, *Gdanscy Ludzie Morza,* 103 ff; *idem,* 'Illness', 97 ff.; *idem,* 'Smierc', 285 ff.; *idem,* 'Tod und Begrabnis der Armen. Ein Beitrag zu Danzigs Alltagsleben im 17. Jh.', *Zeitschrift für Ostforschung,* vol. 41, no. 3, 1992, 321 ff.

53 Maria Bogucka, 'Mentalität der Bürger von Danzig in 16–17. Jh.', *Studia Maritima,* vol. 1, 1978, 64–75.

54 Bogucka, 'Illness', 93

55 See Stanislaw Sokol, *Medycyna w Gdansku w Dobie Odrodzenia (Renaissance Medicine in Danzig),* Wroclaw 1960, *passim.*

56 Kazimierz Kubik, Lech Mokrzecki, *Trzy Wieki Nauki Gdanskiej (Three Centuries of Science in Danzig),* Danzig 1976, 139 ff.

57 Bogucka, 'Illness', 94–5.

58 Simson, *Geschichte,* 182.

59 Bogucka, 'Illness', 96.

60 *ibid.*

61 *ibid.,* 100.

62 *ibid.*

Chapter 10

Poor relief and health care in Scotland, 1575–1710

Rosalind Mitchison

This chapter is of necessity based on very slight material. Little was done in the sixteenth and seventeenth centuries for the sick poor because little or nothing was done for any of the poor in most parts of Scotland, despite the existence of statutes establishing a poor law in the 1570s. It is the failure of social legislation which is the theme of this chapter.

Scotland in the sixteenth century was in cultural, economic and political features indubitably a part of Western Europe. Her society was stratified in ways familiar all over the continent, the divisions between urban communities and rural society the same as elsewhere. She participated in the great cultural developments of the fifteenth- and sixteenth centuries, on the whole belatedly. Her nobles had the same priorities and expenditure patterns as those, for instance, of France. The role of kinship is often stressed in describing her political and social links, but I do not think it marked her out as extraordinary. She was a poor and backward country, of little importance to others except dynastically. The considerable territorial expanse occupied by a small population was one of the reasons why her government was weak: more than half the landmass was occupied by people who paid no attention at all to the demands of the central government and made no financial contribution to it. This area, the Highlands and Western Islands, was effectively independent until conquered by Cromwell in the 1650s. But the government was weak even in the Lowlands. Feudal jurisdictions restricted the area where the king's writ ran. Most of the northern Lowlands lay within one or another of these regalities. The sheriffdoms were hereditary. In much of the country statutes were regarded in the same way as are (a Sicilian once told me) traffic lights in Palermo: advisory rather than mandatory.

The great concern of the sixteenth century with poverty arrived late, if it arrived at all, in Scotland. The Scottish reformation was an issue of power, not of social or religious concern. And it was rather tardy, coming in 1559–60. There was indignation expressed in the Privy Council in 1578 over mobs of poor people at the gates of the royal court in Stirling, 'ane unpleasant and lamentabill spectable' in which the stronger beggars managed to get whatever alms were available at the expense of the 'misterful, suik and impotent'.[1] A few years earlier Parliament had declared that all church organs were to be sold for the poor and that the old Greyfriars convent in Aberdeen should be turned into a hospital – in other words a refuge.[2] These were gestures rather than serious concern for the poor. The early 1570s had been a very disturbed period of political crisis, civil war, English intervention and instability. It was not the time for careful planning of the management of social problems.

So it is rather surprising that the founding statutes of the Old Scottish Poor Law should date from 1575 and 1579.[3] These are the first Acts to combine arrangements for the support of the poor and control of vagabonds, the two essential features of any locally based relief system. The statutes were copies of the English Act of 1572, omitting the orders to set the unemployed at work and making a few minor changes: for instance the roving students denounced for demanding alms were lodged in Scottish universities, not in Oxford or Cambridge. The important difference in the details of the two Scottish Acts was in the authorities who were ordered to take action. In burghs in both cases it was the bailies and provost, in franchises the stewards and bailies, but for the rural 'landward' parishes the first Act, the temporary one, named 'elders and headsmen' – no known lay officials – and the second, the permanent Act, named royal commissioners. There is no evidence that such commissioners were ever appointed.

For the next seventy or so years the main difference between the poor laws of England and Scotland was that in England parishes were gradually managing to work some system of relief while in Scotland, except in a few of the more important burghs, almost nothing was done that had anything to do with obedience to statute law. The Reformed Church had accepted the standard Christian duty towards the poor, and at parish level there were small sums made available for conspicuous need. For instance the published register of the kirk session of St Andrews shows fines being levied on a long list of offences and from 1564 on the money so gained being used occasionally to help the poor and the same is true of Canongate, where the session was established early.[4] These activities were seen as Christian duty, and continued after the poor law statutes had been passed. They were not attempts to make a poor law work, but simply standard expressions of Christian tradition. It seems that the sessions of both parishes spent much more time and paper on disciplining sexual offences than on relief. This is understandable. Poverty was seen as inevitable, but fornication could be stamped on.

How serious was the government of Scotland, in 1575 under the regency of Morton, in 1579 under the personal rule of the twelve-year-old King James VI, in trying to tackle an important social problem? In my opinion it was not serious. This view is based on the failure to organise an administrative system for the Acts in the rural areas, where about 90 per cent of the population lived. The central government could not at this time hope to have any influence in the countryside except through the nobility, until it acquired, bit by bit, some sort of county government which was not hereditary. Sheriffdoms were gradually regained, Justices of the Peace were nominally set up in 1609, but very few were appointed and with limited powers which for the most part they did not exercise. The bishops, whom James VI re-introduced to the church, had some local influence. But county government of any effective kind arrived only with the creation of the Commissioners of Supply in the 1660s.

Meanwhile local government came to be supplied by the Reformed Church through the court structure envisaged in *The First Book of Discipline*. Each parish was to be under a ruling committee of minister and elders, the session. To keep it up to the mark and to decide on major matters there was gradually developed a structure of higher courts, the presbytery, synod and the General Assembly.[5] Eventually the more radical reformers gained enough authority to strengthen the session by making the eldership an office for life. But the model system took time to be established. Even in the Lowlands many northern parishes had not yet got a minister by 1600 and in the Highlands it was not established with any authority until after the rising in 1745. In the 1570s and 80s the concern of the church was to provide educated ministers who could preach. Even through many Catholic priests came into the new church, they were not educated enough to provide a preaching ministry. A new Poor Law Act, that of 1592, reaffirming the earlier ones, marks the time when there could be seen to be a possible rural administration: under Justices and royal commissioners the parishes were to appoint someone to administer the poor law.[6] They did not, of course. They went on with giving out what relief they could afford – not much, for inflation had cut the value of fines. Gradually the system of poor relief run by the sessions as part of Christian duty and supervision by the presbyteries, covered lowland Scotland. But there was very little transfer of resources, whether in money or grain.

There had been little help from the General Assembly, which was engaged in power struggles with the crown: at various times it demanded the bulk of the old endowment of the Catholic Church. Poor relief, as it existed, was based on charitable gifts or fines, not, as the Acts had stipulated, on a rate or 'stent' of land.

The lack of response to the statutes of the 1570s should not surprise. The English poor law of 1572 was effective because it was based on previous activity in many towns, particularly in London. It built on the work of confraternities which had been active even in some rural parishes.[7] They might not have added much to the quantity of relief provided but they had created a recognition of local social responsibility. In Scotland there seem to have been no such organisations. At any rate we have not found their traces. The incorporations or guilds in the burghs had made some effort at mutual aid and support, but they were weak. Rural society appears to have been incorrigibly under the thumb of the nobility. This is not surprising when we remember that the peasantry had no rights in the land they worked.

There were of course pre-Reformation and even post-Reformation endowments, hospitals for instance, where men or women could be nominated to live a semi-monastic life, or leper houses. The purposes of these last was not cure but isolation. It is alleged that the dominant feature of the Edinburgh leper house was a gallows erected beside it to be used on any leper who made contact with townspeople. The city also had a hospital for the poor at the foot of Leith Walk which was turned for a while into a house for children and a House of Industry in which beggars were confined. Later this became a manufactory where the unemployed were put to work.[8] There were numerous small endowments in the northern shires which endured into the seventeenth century as bede houses or hospitals. Probably further research would show these in other parts of the country.[9] The care for the sick in these foundations appears to have been minimal or non-existent.

I have stated in print that nothing was done in response to the Acts of the 1570s until 1649, and recent work has shown that I was wrong. Some of the more important towns tried to get a rate established for the poor, but this was difficult because this type of taxation was unfamiliar. Edinburgh tried to raise a rate in 1575 but gave up after meeting resistance. It tried again in 1580, again unsuccessfully; the crafts claimed that they supported their own members if impoverished. It was only in the plague year of 1584 that it managed to raise a rate, and it was not until 1591 that this became regular.

A few other of the main burghs succeeded in the 1590s in carrying out the legislation, notably St Andrews in 1597 and Perth in 1599. Some other burghs can be seen making some sort of a levy, Aberdeen in 1619, Dundee, the second town of the kingdom, in 1636 and Glasgow at about the same time. It is alleged that Arbroath's support of the poor amounted to a single woman. Aberdeen's was limited by the requirement of regular attendance at church and catechising.[10] Some burghs had charitable legacies left to them to manage for the poor. Some were making plans for sophisticated schemes of welfare and control; Aberdeen in 1636 had plans for a House of Correction, and Edinburgh had established one.[11]

The main relief activity in the countryside, where the bulk of the population lived, was simply the doling out of small sums of money and food. It appears to have been accepted that a peck of oatmeal, weighing about 8.5 pounds, would sustain a not very active adult for a week. Occasionally other needs were noticed, clothing or fuel, and special help as, for instance, when a family's house had been burnt down. Given the scattered pattern of rural settlement there is no reason to believe that all cases of need came to the notice of the sessions. In any case the level of aid given depended on the amount available in the sessions' hands, raised by church collections, fines and occasional legacies. There were also unselective distributions of money by rich landowners at rites of passage. Whatever the statutes said, there was no suggestion of raising a rate in rural areas before 1649. It is worth remembering that Scottish law developed the principle of 'desuetude'. This is the rule that if it could be shown that a statute had not been carried out it lost all force for the future. This doctrine is one of the reasons for the large amount of systematic misrepresentation in accounts of the Scottish Poor Law.

The inadequate base of rural poor relief was shown up sharply after the harvest failure of 1622. The level of destitution needed support on a scale which the spare cash of a needy peasantry could not supply; in other words it needed to tap the surplus which went in rent to the landowner. It did not get it. Midsummer 1623 the Privy Council, alarmed, sent out an Act (order) to the sheriffs, justices, bailies and regalities, landowners and ministers of the shires, to assess what the local need before the next harvest would be, to buy in grain and 'stent' the inhabitants to pay for it. Ministers were to report the number of poor in their parishes. A further order covered the arrest of vagrants, their imprisonment and support, paid for by a stent on landowners.

The replies from the shires dribbled in from August onwards, and were not very satisfactory. While some, for instance Perthshire, indicated willingness to raise funds and distribute grain, and others, Renfrewshire, Mearns, Stirlingshire and West Lothian, were fairly cooperative, many replies were vague and general: Berwickshire promised merely to do what was possible. Some show a real recognition of the problem of relief: Selkirkshire stated that there was a lack of employment. One of the most dilatory answers, sent in November, was from East Lothian, the richest agricultural area in Scotland: a flat refusal to act. It picked holes in the authority of the Council's act and the proposed system of raising funds to support beggars and stated that being expected to act was 'toylsome and troublesome . . . importing nethair credeit nor benefeit', and adding 'every contribution is odious and smellis of ane taxatioun'. Those who dominated Scottish rural society had in no way accepted the authority of the statutes in the matter of raising a rate.[12]

Though assessment for relief had not yet been accepted by those who would have to pay, the church was moving towards more systematic aid to the poor from voluntary sources. Parishes began to keep regular pension lists of their poor. But the regular pensions were not enough to live on, and the poor were expected to beg as well, and might be given badges to show that the activity was approved.[13]

It was in 1649 that some approximation to the poor law became effective in most lowland parishes. At this moment the covenanting party in the church had seized power: the aristocracy was in eclipse, some of it in prison in England, others doing penance in church for the wrong political decisions. Parliament, excluding the aristocracy from all office bearing, passed a realistic Act accepting the role of voluntary support as the norm but empowering parishes to rate their landowners when more was needed, and handing over relief in the countryside to the church.[14] At last we can see the poor law working in most of lowland Scotland.

After the Restoration it continued to work. Grain prices were low and until the mid 1690s supplies were adequate. Parishes ran a minimal level of relief to keep people from starving, mostly by money doles. Names can be found on the list of pensioners for several years, showing that people were surviving in poverty. There are frequent references to legacies for the poor, though often parishes found these difficult to extract from the kin of the donors. Altogether by the 1690s relief was working at a low level in most lowland areas in prosperous times, and was elastic in the concept of the needs that should be met. Parishes would provide wet nurses for motherless infants or families with twins. They seem to have been particularly generous in care for the insane, giving money for food, clothes and someone to wash and clean.

It should not surprise us that most of this activity was by means of money. An economically backward country can be highly monetised. In Scotland most rents and many wages were still paid in kind but a surprisingly large amount of money did circulate: it was not unusual for landowners to borrow from their own tenants. The pastoral economy developing in the Borders was the most highly monetised part of Scotland.[15]

The famine of the 1690s, four years in five of inadequate harvests, showed the limitations of the poor relief system. Of the parishes for which records survive, 229 in number, about a fifth were able to raise money on assessment from their landowners. Many of those which managed to do this did it only in the last year of the bad times under particularly heavy pressure from the Privy Council and the organs of county government. The loss of life in the famine was probably over 10 per cent of the population, more in the north. The priority with which the poor law was normally worked, that is to keep those who could not keep themselves from starving, was confirmed as appropriate to the state of economy and society.

Things became very different in the eighteenth century. Land-owners, though not relishing assessment, were anxious to be seen making generous gifts to the poor. There is evidence of effective county activity, in bad times the buying of grain abroad and offering it under price to the sessions. With the foundation of the early infirmaries and the medical schools, parishes could make arrangements for their sick.

But back before 1700, with so little support from the landowners, what sort of medical relief can be expected? Edinburgh, the only town then that can be considered a city in status, size and width of activities, can be seen to be making some limited aid specifically for the sick. In 1578 the town paid a surgeon nine pounds three and fourpence Scots, about £1 sterling, for drugs, plasters and medicaments to the poor. The sum was about what a well off merchant would pay for medical services to his household.[16] There is no mention of medical relief again in the published excerpts of the Edinburgh burgh records until the 1620s, but from 1627 the city regularly appointed a surgeon to care for the poor and paid his expenses.[17] In June 1645 it paid 100 pounds Scots a month to a physician to care for the poor 'inclosed or infected' by the plague. The medicament side of medical relief rose steadily. In 1674 it was fifteen pounds thirteen and fourpence Scots. In 1676 the burgh council decided that it would not pay for any treatment which it had not directly authorised and had costed in advance by a bailie. In 1694 it had a new idea for cutting the cost: the surgeon appointed to the poor was promised the bodies of those beggars who died in the Correction House and of all foundlings who died while still at the breast. At least one public dissection a year was expected. But the scheme did not work. Four years later, a surgeon was given 400 pounds Scots because the ruling had provided completely ineffectual. It seems that the beggars in the Correction House had made or threatened trouble.[18]

The first year for which we have detailed accounts of what the treatment of the poor consisted of is 1710. Ninety-four patients then received treatment. In some cases there was frequent attention, in one case on consecutive days. Purges, oils, plaster, gargles and bleeding, bone setting and amputation were applied. There seems to have been an undesirable amount of mercury ointment in use. That at least one course of treatment was successful is shown by the appearance of a woman having a leg amputated, who six months later is provided with a 'timber leg'. The total cost that year was 433 pounds four shillings Scots, or £36.2s sterling.[19]

Similar activity, starting later, can be found in Glasgow, which in the seventeenth century was moving rapidly to the position of the second town in Scotland. The first grant for medical aid to the poor in the published burgh records came in 1627–8. In the 1650s repayment of surgeon's expenses in supplying drugs to the poor became regular. In 1668 seven poor persons were treated for

twenty-seven pounds fourteen shillings; in 1673 the charges had
grown to sixty-one pounds sixteen shillings, and in 1679 to seventy-
nine pounds ten shillings and fourpence. As in Edinburgh, the town
council attempted to check the upward trend by insisting that a
bailie had to authorise all prescriptions. There is an interesting entry
in the accounts for 1700 for the treatment of a man who had broken
his arm and dislocated his knee in a fire. For thirty pounds Scots
these were mended and he was given 'medicaments external and
internal' for bruises and the spitting of blood. I have no idea what,
among the drugs then in use, could have been serviceable for these
injuries. In 1652 a woman had been 'cured' in ten weeks of
treatment after a soldier had struck the 'knap' of her elbow. Again
what degree of cure could be delivered is unclear.[20]

A trawl through the archives of other burghs might well produce
other references to payments for treatment in the later seventeenth
century. The kirk session register of St Andrews shows the parish
organising medical aid in 1599, and there were bigger and more
prosperous towns than this.[21]

Even rural parishes can be found to be paying for somewhat
ambiguous forms of aid in the second half of the century. For
instance in East Lothian in 1695, Spott, a parish supporting a
crippled orphan boy, heard that the woman paid to look after him
would not do so when he had an attack of diarrhoea without more
payment: she was given an extra pound Scots and the boy was given
a wheelbarrow in which he could be wheeled about to beg. The same
parish in 1691 gave money to 'a poor boy that had had his foot cut
off'. In 1700 Yester, also in East Lothian, paid out one pound ten
shillings Scots 'for aile to Janet Burn when she was sick'. Lintrathen
in 1696 made a special collection for a man who had had his leg
'cut' by a physician. In Lunan, 1697, a payment was made to a man
who could not pay the doctor's fee for a stone operation to his son,
and Guthrie paid for the maintenance of a woman in Forfar who was
sent there for cure of a cancer on her lip.[22] These entries have a
bearing on health but do not show the parishes directly involved in
care. The practical arrangements were made by the sufferer or their
kin, not by the parish. Outside the bigger towns there is no
evidence of any parish linkages with the medical profession or any
regular payment for medical attention.

It seems clear that men with medical or surgical qualifications
were rare outside the large towns. The surviving records of the poll
taxes of the 1690s show that Edinburgh was plentifully supplied

with professional aid: nineteen apothecaries, twenty-three surgeons and thirty-three doctors of medicine in 1694.[23] Glasgow had enough to maintain a 'faculty' of physicians and surgeons. Aberdeen had four apothecary surgeons and three physicians. There was a single physician in St Andrews. The testaments for the Dumfries commissariot court give the names of two surgeons existing in that city in the years 1624–1700, and doubtless other commissariots would yield a similar number. The area for which we have full poll tax material, Aberdeenshire, shows no medical men in the landward area of the shire.[24] All varieties of medical men figure in the wealthier parts of society, and presumably were there to serve people equally well endowed. Poll tax records may not be complete: failure to pay this tax is not confined to the twentieth century. And the commissariot's coverage had gaps too. But it seems likely that there was no professional medical or surgical aid available in the landward parishes where the bulk of the people lived.

Lack of medical aid for most of the country should be seen only as a small part of the shortcomings of the early poor law in Scotland. Simply there was very little available in aid before 1649 and even after that date not enough to cope with the level of need in an emergency. If support was not available when a third of the people in a parish were in danger of starvation, it is useless to expect that there would be adequate help for a man who broke his leg. The question that needs to be asked is not why was there so little medical aid but why so little was done altogether in the way of relief.

First of all we must recognise that Scotland, until the eighteenth century, was a conspicuously poor country. She had a scattered population farming the patches of good soil, some of it very good, in an incompetent, traditional manner in an uncertain and often hostile climate. Her exports were mostly raw materials or very crude industrial products. The only high quality item here was an entirely natural product, coal. In the sixteenth- and early seventeenth centuries when England was diversifying her textile industries, Scotland was producing only low-quality woollens for export. There was not much wealth around, and what there was was taken over by the landowning class.

Until the mid-seventeenth century the church as a national institution had done little for the poor. There does not seem to have been much in the way of medieval religious support of the poor, which is understandable when we remember that by the late fifteenth century 87 per cent of Scottish parishes had been impropriated for some religious foundation or other, a monastery or collegiate church. To participate in the great ecclesiastical and cultural movements of Europe, Scotland had seen her parishes robbed. That part of the tithe which was notionally for the poor simply was not available. Then in their turn the monasteries had been robbed by the kings who had placed them in *commendam* (as benefices) so that their illegitimate sons could be handsomely provided for. After the Reformation the church was struggling to get back lands and tithes, but this was a political issue between General Assembly and the King and Parliament, and no attention was paid in the later sixteenth century to making the poor law effective.

It is my impression that in most of Western Europe the effective areas of poor relief were the cities. This seems true for Italy, France and Spain. England appears exceptional in having created a working system of poor relief in rural areas. Scotland in the sixteenth- and seventeenth centuries was one of the less urbanised parts of Europe. By whatever concentration of population you take as an indicator of urban life she comes out low, though not as low as Scandinavia or Eastern Europe.[25] Until medical qualifications became more common, medical aid could be found only in towns, and people in the country had either to do without or to manage a difficult journey on bad roads. Even in the last days of the old Scottish Poor Law, the 1840s, many parishes had no better medical aid than a medicine chest kept by the minister.

The Scottish poor law long failed to work because landed society refused to work it. In so far as any relief existed outside a few leading towns, it existed as independent provision by the church. So it is to landed society that we should look for explanation of the poor law's failure to operate. The great landowners in Scotland were simply not in the habit of taking orders from the crown: they regarded the Stewarts as merely a jumped up family of status similar to their own, very similar, for almost all the important nobility could take their ancestry back to one or other of the confused marriages of Robert II, the first royal Stewart. Where the great men led the lesser landowners were bound to follow: the class of lairds was not strong enough to stand up for itself until the eighteenth century. Landowners had been grabbing the property of the church well before the Reformation. After this event they had been granted more church lands and tithes, but great insecurity hung about these grants. Any landed family which had to play a part in politics feared annihilation: all politics was a game of snakes and ladders. Statutes existed which the monarch was rarely powerful enough to enforce, but which could be used against some noble who played his cards badly. The reign of Charles I and James VI show instances of families thus destroyed. In particular the entire nobility feared that the crown might revoke gifts of lands or tithes: the result would be, if not penury, at least inability to maintain the standard of living expected of European nobles. The nobility was quite right to be afraid, as Charles I's Act of Revocation showed. In the end what was worked out under this Act was not a total despoliation of the nobility, but it took several years for this to become apparent. In such a state of insecurity it would be surprising if the great landowners felt any need to provide for the equally insecure lower end of society. The lesser landowners, the men who mattered in every parish, were also insecure, subject to pressures from the nobility, at risk of being obliged to enter into some band or agreement or subject to some feud. The eighteenth-century achievements of making the poor law work at least in the Lowlands was the work of a society freed from these sources of insecurity, by men with sure rent rolls. But things had been very different before the Great Rebellion.

I have recently been working in the field of the mid-nineteenth century poor law, and what I have seen there obliges me to point out that this chapter is asking the wrong question. In the 1840s, as a Royal Commission painstakingly revealed, and what many people must have already known, the legal obligations on landowners to fund relief where needed were simply not being carried out. Landowners in many rural parishes not only evaded setting rates but gave very little in charity.[26] Where relief existed it was grossly inadequate. Anyone who inquired around systematically could have found this out, yet until a crisis in a major industrial town blew up, nothing was done. And this was in an advanced industrial country with excellent means of communication. We should not be asking why societies ignore the needs of the poor and fail to provide relief, but why in some periods do some of them manage to do something about it.

NOTES

1   *Register of the Privy Council of Scotland* (hereafter *RPCS*), vol. III, 1578–85, ed. P. Hume Brown, Edinburgh 1901, 137; 'misterful' means impoverished or necessitous.

2   *RPCS*, vol. II, 1569–78, ed. P. Hume Brown, Edinburgh 1900, 435.

3   *Acts of the Parliaments of Scotland* (hereafter APS), 12 volumes, Edinburgh 1814–75, vol. III, 87, 139. (1575 and 1579).

4   D. H. Fleming (ed.) *Register of the Minister, Elders and Deacons of St Andrews, 1559–1600*, 2 vols, Scottish History Society, Edinburgh 1889 and 1890, 233 ff. A. B. Calderwood (ed.) *The Buik of the Kirk of the Canagait, 1564–67*, Scottish Record Society, Edinburgh 1961, 3 ff.

5   James Kirk, *The Second Book of Discipline*, Edinburgh 1980, 102–14.

6   *APS*, III, 576.

7   E. M. Leonard, *The Early History of Poor Relief*, Cambridge 1900; Margery McIntosh, 'Local Responses to the Poor in Late Mediaeval and Tudor England', *Continuity and Change*, III (1986) 209–43.

8   Robert Thin, 'The Old Infirmary and Other Hospitals', *The Buik of the Old Edinburgh Club*, xv, 1927, 135–63; *Extracts from the Records of the Merchant Guild of Stirling A.D. 1592–1846*, Scottish Burgh Record Society, Stirling 1916, 21; record of a gift to the town's hospital, 1592.

9   Marguerite Wood, 'The Domestic Affairs of the Burgh', *The Buik of the Old Edinburgh Club*, vol. xix, 1933, 11–154. J. M. McPherson, *The Kirk's Care of the Poor*, Aberdeen, 1945, 127–41, 163–73.

10 J. H. Goodare, 'Parliament and Society in Scotland, 1563–1603', Edinburgh University PhD thesis 1989, Chapter 8.

11 *Extracts from the Records of the Burgh of Edinburgh, 1626–41* (hereafter *Edinburgh Extracts*), vol. vii, ed. Marguerite Wood, Scottish Burgh Record Society, Edinburgh 1926, 172, 3 February 1636.

12 *RPCS*, XIII, 1622–7, ed. D. Masson, Edinburgh 1895, 357–60, 289–90, 805–834.

13 e.g. H. Paton, *The Session Book of Dundonald*, Edinburgh 1936, privately published, 400 ff.

14 *APS*, VI, ii, 220.

15 R. A. Dodgshon, *Land and Society in Early Scotland*, Oxford 1981, Chapter 6. I. D. and K. A. Whyte, 'Debt and Credit, Poverty and Prosperity in a Seventeenth-Century Scottish Rural Community', in Rosalind Mitchison and Peter Roebuck eds, *Economy and Society in Scotland and Ireland, 1500–1939*, Edinburgh 1988, 70–80.

16 *Edinburgh Extracts*, vol. IV, 1573–89, Edinburgh 1882, 535, January 1589, and 436, September 1585.

17 *Edinburgh Extracts*, vol. VII, 1626–41, Edinburgh 1938, 21 February 1627.

18 *Edinburgh Extracts*, 1665–80, (1950) June 1645; February 1674 and 265, April 1676; vol. XII, Helen Armet (ed) 161, October 1694 and 231, June 1698.

19 My thanks are due to Doctor Helen Dingwall who kindly gave me this material. The original is in the Royal College of Surgeons, Edinburgh.

20 *Extracts from the Records of the Burgh of Glasgow*, vol. 1, 1573–1642, Scottish Burgh Record Society, Glasgow 1876, 479; vol. III, 1663–90, (1905) 16, July 1663: 28, April 1664; 104, April 1668:

167, May 1673; vol. IV, 1691–1717, (1906) 308, September 1700; vol. II, 1630–62, (1881) 242, September 1652.

21 D. H. Fleming (ed.) *St Andrews*, vol. 2, 82, 28 February 1597.

22 Scottish Record Office, CH2/377/2; CH2/333/2; CH2/243/1; CH2/253/6; CH2.535/1. These last three parishes are all in Angus, but similar entries can be found for other areas.

23 H. M. Dingwall, *Late Seventeenth-Century Edinburgh*, Aldershot 1994, 289–93.

24 *List of Pollable Persons in the Shire of Aberdeen*, New Spalding Club, Aberdeen 1844, vol. 2, 632; D. Macfarlane, 'St Andrews in the 1690s from the Poll Tax', MA thesis, Edinburgh University Department of Economic and Social History, MA thesis, 1981; Francis J. Grant (ed) *Commissariot Record of Dumfries: Register of Testaments 1625–1801*, Scottish Record Society, Edinburgh 1902. Stirling burgh records refer to an 'insufficient' surgeon in 1509, *Extracts . . . Royal Burgh of Stirling*, Scottish Burgh Record Society, Glasgow 1887.

25 I. D. Whyte, 'Population Mobility in Early Modern Scotland', in R. A. Houston and I. D. Whyte, *Scottish Society, 1500–1800*, Cambridge 1988, 43–4.

26 *Parliamentary Papers 1844*, vols XX–XXII.

Chapter 11

Hospitals, workhouses and the relief of the poor in early modern London

Paul Slack

Praising the new naval hospital at Greenwich in 1728, the architect Nicholas Hawksmoor declared that such institutions were one of the necessary means of 'rectifying the irregular and ill management of the police of great cities'.[1] By that he meant that hospitals were both a testimony to enlightened civic policies and a mechanism for instituting and preserving social order. They had admirably fulfilled both functions in Louis XIV's Paris; now they might do the same in Georgian London. Aspirations of this kind were by no means new in London, however. For two centuries before 1728, hospitals had been visualised as institutions which might not only express charitable instincts, relieve the poor, and protect public health, but in doing all those things bring about civic regulation and civic regeneration.

The story is a large and sometimes convoluted one. In what follows I propose to try to highlight what seem to me its main features by describing five different episodes in its chronological development. Each exemplifies a different approach to charity and civic welfare. Each had international origins or consequences, or both, and hence has something to contribute to the theme of this volume. And each is of historical interest in its own right. I have called these episodes royal, civic, metropolitan, baroque and voluntary.[2]

THE ROYAL EPISODE

There were, of course, already a number of hospitals in London in the fifteenth century, perhaps as many as thirty, depending on how one defines them. Some were products of the wave of religious foundations of the twelfth and thirteenth centuries, some more recent erections, commonly almshouses like those founded by Sir

Richard Whittington in 1424.[3] In 1505 Henry VII added to their number by embarking on his own great work of mercy, the Savoy Hospital. Designed 'to receive and lodge nightly one hundred poor folks', it was an asylum and hospice for beggars, travellers and pilgrims, and it seems, despite its size, wholly traditional in purpose.

Yet the organisation of the Savoy was based on that of the hospital of Santa Maria Nuova in Florence, whose statutes the King had examined; and its cruciform shape looked back to the Great Hospital in Milan. It introduced to England the movement for hospital reform which had improved the management and revived the social purpose of these institutions in fifteenth-century Italy; and it was one example of Italian influence on English social policy at this time, of which another was Cardinal Wolsey's founding of the College of Physicians in 1518, soon after the Savoy was completed. Intended to be matched by similar huge foundations in Coventry and York, the Savoy might have set a trend.[4] We have only to look ahead, to Cardinal Pole's and Bishop Bonner's encouragement of gifts to such foundations in the reign of Mary, to see that England might have taken part in that Catholic new philanthropy of the sixteenth century which produced both institutions and fraternities directed to the relief of the disadvantaged and the dispossessed.

The English Reformation, the dissolution of religious orders and fraternities and the confiscation of their property, including many hospitals, put a stop in the 1530s and 1540s to any such prospect. It now became a matter of saving what could be saved from the wreckage of traditional charity; and the consequent *tabula rasa* made the rulers of London – like those of other reformed or reforming European cities – define their most urgent priorities and rethink their charitable and civic priorities. In 1538 the citizens petitioned the king for the restoration to them of the old hospitals of St Bartholomew's and St Thomas's, not, they hastened to say, for 'priests, canons and monks carnally living', but for 'the miserable people lying in every street, offending every clean person passing by the way, with their filthy and nasty savours'. It was partly a matter of Christian charity – 'the relief of Christ's very images' in the streets, and partly a matter of civic necessity – 'for the avoiding of the great infections and other inconveniences' they might cause if not properly housed.[5]

Henry VIII's response was slow and partial – the grant to the City of St Bartholomew's in 1544 and of the Greyfriars and other religious property in 1546. But it was as pious in tone as the bequest of his father. The buildings should be used for the traditional works of mercy, reinstituted now 'according to the primitive pattern'. Edward VI completed the process, giving the City his father's old palace at Bridewell, and the landed endowments of the Savoy (though not its buildings), and enabling five hospitals to be restored or founded, and ultimately united as 'the hospitals of Edward the Sixth of England'. If the royal input continued, however, it was a contribution more in name than in substance. For the initiative came from the City. The united royal hospitals were the product of prolonged debate in committees of London aldermen and common councillors, discussing new 'plats' or models for welfare reform, and deciding in the end on their own ideal project, 'a perfect platform of a common wealth'.[6] In effect, the royal hospitals belong to a second, civic episode.

THE CIVIC EPISODE

The five hospitals each had a different purpose: St Bartholomew's for the sick, St Thomas's for the old and impotent, Christ's Hospital in the old Greyfriars for the 'virtuous education and bringing up' of orphan children and foundlings, Bethlehem Hospital for lunatics, and Bridewell for employing the idle poor in 'sciences profitable to the comonweal'.[7] Through their joint management, the five institutions were also intended to provide a central organisation which would receive charitable collections (and later compulsory assessments) from the parishes of the City, and redistribute them where necessary to deserving poor householders, especially those burdened with large numbers of children. The whole scheme was one for the central focusing of charity on secularly defined and carefully discriminated social targets. As such, it was not unlike the blueprints for centralised welfare institutions in several European Reformed cities.

It is unfortunate, therefore, that the sources do not allow us to specify the precise chains of influence from the continent to England which lay behind the London programme. Some links may have been provided by the congregations of Dutch and French Protestant refugees in Edwardian London, but their influence seems to have been slender at this stage. Bishop Ridley of London certainly provided an intellectual gloss to the whole scheme which he had perhaps learned from evangelical theologians and churches. More obvious, and probably more powerful, however, were the constant contacts between the Merchant Adventurers of London and the cities of the Low Countries to which they exported cloth. Powerful figures in the early history of the hospitals, like the aldermen and Merchant Adventurers, Richard Gresham and Rowland Hill, would certainly have known about contemporary developments in social welfare in Bruges, and possibly also in Ypres. The rulers of London were part of a North-European mercantile network which must have had an impact on civic as well as economic policy in England.

Yet one part of the London apparatus was unique: Bridewell, 'the house of labour and occupations', founded in 1552, where the poor should be set to work. A hospital specifically and solely for employment appears to have no parallel in the many published tracts on social welfare of the period, which often stressed the need for labour but visualised its place outside institutions, not in a purpose-built hospital. Neither, so far as I am aware, did Bridewell have any precedent in reality in other European cities or states, which commonly dealt with their beggars in other ways: by simply banishing them from cities, or employing them in the galleys. Bridewell's roots lay rather in English circumstances: in the failure of the statutes of 1536, 1547 and 1552 which founded the English poor law effectively to combat idleness by setting beggars and the unemployed to useful labour; and in the peculiar economic conditions of the 1540s, when debasement of the coinage produced unprecedented inflation, and stimulated public awareness of economic problems, including the need for new industries and employment. Its founders promised to employ the poor on new kinds of metalwork, for example, and on the production of goods such as caps of the same quality as those imported from abroad.[8] A 'house of occupations' seemed an answer to a range of current economic and social problems. Whatever its particular English origins, however, Bridewell had an international influence, spawning offspring first in many other English cities and then all over Europe, particularly after the opening of the 'house of discipline' in Amsterdam in 1596.[9] England's first original contribution to European welfare strategies was not compulsory taxation for the poor, the poor rate, though this was the second. The first, and the one most widely copied, was the workhouse.

The poor rate did, however, have an important effect on the future development of the London hospital system, for it decisively undermined one of its chief purposes: central control of poor relief over the entire city. From the beginning the one hundred or so parishes of the City of London had been reluctant to transfer the whole of their charitable collections for the poor to a central treasury at Christ's Hospital; and the national poor law of 1598 strengthened their hand by making the parish, with its overseers, the essential unit for collecting rates and dispensing outdoor relief. For a time following the Poor Act of 1572 Christ's Hospital continued to receive part of parish rates, but after 1598 even this effort at central control ceased.[10] At the same time, Bridewell itself was being undermined. There was an inherent conflict between the two divergent roles as conceived by its founders: the first, to provide employment and training in useful trades; the second, simply to cleanse the streets from rogues, prostitutes and undesirables, to 'punish sin', in the words of the hospital's Elizabethan historian John Howes. The second role was naturally easier to fulfil than the first. By the 1580s Bridewell had become a lockup for petty offenders, and hence, like the old Savoy at the same time, it could be castigated as 'a nursery of rogues, thieves, idle and drunken persons'.[11] It was far from the ideal of its founders.

Contemporaries were aware of the problem, of course. Following long discussion with a Privy Council equally alarmed by poverty in the city, new orders in 1582 returned to the ideal that Bridewell should be for the poor's 'reformation and not for perpetual servitude'. They proposed the reintroduction of a host of useful trades: shoemaking, nailmaking, spinning of woollen and linen yarn, wire-drawing, pinmaking, knife-making, the new crafts of bay- and felt-making, and the manufacture of tennis balls.[12] In the 1620s, Alderman Sir Thomas Middleton, member of the Dutch Church at Austin Friars, proposed wholly new workhouses for small groups of parishes where the poor would be employed on hemp and other useful trades. None of these suggestions had any major effect.[13]

Meanwhile, the growth of the city presented new problems and aggravated old ones. A population of perhaps 100,000 in the mid-sixteenth century had become one of 200,000 by 1600 and 355,000 by 1640. The royal hospitals, which handled 4,000 people a year at the beginning of the seventeenth century, could not cope with the social fallout. Moreover, the built-up area was from the 1580s visibly expanding beyond that controlled by the Corporation of the City. In 1630, when a minor outbreak of plague coincided with dearth and economic depression, the Privy Council itself had to act as, in effect, a Greater London Council, trying to coordinate poor relief in the City and in the growing East and West Ends and the streets beyond Southwark, which fell under the jurisdiction of the justices of the peace of Middlesex and Surrey.[14] Prolonged discussion and dispute between Council and City about the problem of the suburbs produced no agreement before 1640: the City declined any invitation to extend its jurisdiction to new areas where social problems were concentrated. But the metropolitan issue was now firmly on the agenda, and though never satisfactorily resolved, it helped to shape projects over the next generation, and hence what might be called the metropolitan episode.

THE METROPOLITAN EPISODE

The centrepiece of the metropolitan episode was the London Corporation of the Poor: a separate legal entity alongside the Corporation of the City of London, set up by parliamentary ordinance in 1647 and further refined by Act of Parliament in 1649.[15] Though separate from the municipality, its governors overlapped with those of the City: the Lord Mayor was *ex officio* President, a number of the Aldermen were members of it, and its other governing 'Assistants' were, in 1647, to be appointed by the Common Council of London, and, in 1649, to be directly elected by the various City wards. This new corporate body had three purposes, all arising out of past experience. The first was to provide, once again, the centralised control of social welfare which the royal hospitals had once promised. The second was to organise new workhouses of the kind Middleton had in mind. The third – and the legal purpose of incorporation – was to allow the new organisation to receive and manage charitable benefactions.

What the London Corporation of the Poor did not have was authority outside the boundaries of the old city. Yet that is what some of its sponsors had wanted. It had been discussed first in the City in 1641 and 1642, with that limitation firmly in place; but when the subject was taken up again in 1645 it was at the suggestion of pressure groups with wider ends in view. There was a petition for the Corporation, supported in part by merchants to the 'western parts', the colonial merchants who were then rising to power in the City, including Nicholas Corselis, a member of the Dutch Church at Austin Friars.[16] But the campaign seems to have been organised by Samuel Hartlib, the German emigré at the centre of a group of writers seeking to bring about a total reformation of knowledge and public welfare, a 'Great Instauration' on Baconian principles, in an England set free by political revolution.

The Hartlib group contributed to extraordinary twice-weekly public meetings organised by the Lord Mayor for 'all such as are well-affected to so pious and charitable a work'; and they published tracts in support of the new Corporation. One of them, by Leonard Lee, saw the need for an organisation supervising social welfare over the whole metropolis, including Westminster, Middlesex and urban Surrey, where 'most of the poor do live'.[17] Another, *The Poor Man's Friend* (1649), by Rice Bush, proposed what amounted to a complete welfare state: surveys of the poor in London and beyond; free medical services for the poor and free education for their children; stocks of material on which they could draw for work at home as well as in institutions; encouragement to the cultivation of wastes and the growing of hemp, both to set the poor on work making ropes and nets, and to benefit the fisheries and the navy. Much of this, of course, was utopian, but that is part of its interest. Hartlib had a total vision incorporating projects and achievements drawn from other countries as well as England: from the clean streets freed from beggars and paupers of cities in the Low Countries, to the teaching hospitals of Paris and (a little later) its *Hôpital-Général*. Thus informed, London was to be a model both for a national reformation and for the erection of the 'Kingdom of Christ' throughout the world.

In the event these aspirations were cut down to size. Bush was one of those piloting the legislation for the Corporation of the Poor of 1647 and 1649 through parliament, and he had to make concessions, including the important one limiting the Corporation's territorial jurisdiction to the old city. The 1647 ordinance had a clause permitting similar corporations in boroughs or counties which wanted them, but none volunteered. Bush and Corselis were also among the governing Assistants of the London Corporation after 1649, and they may then have achieved some of their ends. There was a register of the poor; children (up to eighty at a time) were sent to the new workhouse to be taught as well as employed; up to 1,000 adults were set to work in their own homes.[18] Although the official records of the Corporation do not survive, it looks as if more was achieved than had ever been accomplished under the aegis of Bridewell or the various schemes for its reform.

The London Corporation of the Poor collapsed with the return of the Stuarts in 1660 and the restoration to Charles II of the royal properties which the Corporation had occupied; but the metropolitan issue, and the proposed solution, did not die with it. In 1661 parliament considered a bill for a single London Corporation of the Poor for the whole area within the bills of mortality, that is, virtually the whole built-up area, with no fewer than 200 Assistants, Corselis among them. There was another bill constituting Corporations of the Poor 'in the several cities and counties within the kingdom'. Both were dropped in the House of Lords, however. What came out were the clauses in the Act of Settlement of 1662 which simply authorised the erection of Corporations in London and Westminster, and separate ones in urban Middlesex and Surrey.[19]

Nevertheless, workhouses and work schemes, and especially those training children, which had been an essential part of the programme of the Hartlib group, remained central to public discussion of the poor of the metropolis. A Corporation of the Poor for Middlesex was founded under the 1662 Act, with a workhouse at Clerkenwell which was much admired by visitors including Samuel Pepys, who applauded, as Hartlib might have done, 'the many pretty works, and the little children employed, everyone to do something'. The London Quakers, who had a flax-spinning project for their poor from about 1677, looked back to earlier projects, and so did the Socinian, Thomas Firmin, who was employing and training poor children in St Botolph's Aldersgate at about the same time. The London Corporation of the Poor, in abeyance since 1660, was itself revived in 1698, under the aegis of Firmin's patron the great Whig magnate Sir Robert Clayton, when parliaments after the Glorious Revolution again sought a national reformation and saw institutions for the reform and regulation of the poor as an essential part of it.[20]

Yet there was no single controlling hand in later Stuart London to coordinate its policies and provision for social welfare. Sectarian and political divisions prevented that, and encouraged instead a proliferation of different mechanisms. Clayton's revived Whig Corporation of the Poor, with its new workhouse in Bishopsgate, was opposed, and in effect emasculated, by interests in the parishes, many of them Tory in political affiliation and all deeply antagonistic to the reintroduction of anything like central municipal control. The old royal hospitals responded to threats from new corporations by publicising their continuing utility, but they were divided among themselves by the different political complexions of their governing bodies, a largely Whig St Thomas's being set against a Tory St Bartholomew's in the 1680s, for example. While Christ's Hospital began to raise its social profile and the status of its clientele with the new Mathematical School founded in 1673, and a school for girls set up at Hertford in the 1690s, Anglican divines, alarmed by threats from Dissent and Popery, were embarking on their own panacea for social ills, charity schools.[21]

Like the Quaker employment schemes, most of these projects owed something to the legacy of Hartlib and his fellow projectors. But they were testimony also to a plurality of rival institutions and organisations all claiming a hand in social welfare in late seventeenth-century London. Its most dramatic manifestation was a competitive craze for building, which created what seems to me to merit the designation of the baroque episode.

THE BAROQUE EPISODE

A new era for London's hospitals opened with the Great Fire of London of 1666, or rather with the subsequent rebuilding. It is perhaps a sign of their low status in the 1660s that the royal hospitals had no special place in the splendid vistas which Christopher Wren planned for the new city or in John Evelyn's proposed piazzas, unlike churches, the Guildhall or the Exchange. But rebuilding gave them the chance to remedy this, to enhance their prestige and demonstrate their wealth and social purpose with new constructions which should be 'for use and charity'.[22]

Of the royal hospitals, only Bridewell and Christ's had been burned in the fire. Both were reconstructed on their original courtyard plans, the first with help from the coal duties voted by parliament, since it now counted as a prison, the second thanks to gifts from benefactors, Robert Clayton chief among them. But Clayton's example led the rival governors of Bethlehem to undertake something much more remarkable: the erection in 1676 of a completely new Bedlam on an elongated site, given by the City, on the southern edge of Moorfields, with the City wall behind it. Designed by Robert Hooke, architect of the new College of Physicians, its site, plan and elevation gave it light, air and a grandeur which influenced most later hospital buildings.

So brave, so neat, so sweet, it does appear,
Makes one half-mad to be a lodger there

says a contemporary celebration.[23]

The new Bedlam, which proved such an attraction to visitors for
a century and more, may tell us something about changing
sensibilities. Like the contemporary interest in the education of
young children, a sensitivity to insanity suggests an extension of
charitable benevolence beyond the worthy elderly paupers and
labouring poor householders who had been its chief targets for a
century. 'What objects then more claim our charity', asks the same
author, 'Than those that know not their own misery?' But the new
extended charity was certainly to be known and to be displayed:
advertised in engravings of the City with Bedlam prominent in the
foreground, just as some contemporary prints of Paris were
dominated by Louis XIV's military hospital of the *Invalides*, begun
in 1670.[24]

The example of the *Invalides* brought Charles II into the game,
with a hospital for another target of public benevolence. English
kings had, of course, long faced the problem of housing maimed
soldiers and military veterans, and had used part of the much
mangled Savoy Hospital for the purpose since the 1620s. In the
Second Dutch War of the 1660s the King's Commissioners for Sick
and Wounded had contemplated requisitioning almshouses and
hospitals throughout the kingdom for them; but a national survey,
undertaken in 1665, had shown that it would have cost more effort
than it was worth: the eighty-nine institutions for which returns
survive housed only seven inmates each on average.[25] In 1680,
however, the King's Lieutenant in Ireland, Ormonde, showed the
way, copying the *Invalides* with the building of Kilmainham
Hospital, Dublin; and in 1682, thanks to Stephen Fox and
deductions from the grants for soldiers' pay, Chelsea Hospital could
be begun.[26] Though not completed until 1691, it was Charles II's
version of Henry VII's great work of charity at the Savoy, and the
precursor of the even grander Greenwich Hospital of William III
and Anne. The two together were the royal contribution to the new
fashion for monumental embodiments of public ideals.

That was not the end. Chelsea and Greenwich stimulated
building elsewhere: at St Thomas's where Clayton was again lavish
with effort and money in the 1690s and 1700s; and in the rival
Tory-dominated St Bartholomew's, whose governors were at last

busy with their own rebuilding in the later 1720s. In 1724 Thomas Guy, a major benefactor of St Thomas's, left his fortune for the erection next door of a new hospital for the incurably sick and infirm which was intended to rival 'the endowment of kings'.[27] This was plainly competitive conspicuous expenditure on a grand scale. But it could be defended, as it was by Hawksmoor, whom I cited at the beginning of this paper. For him new hospitals were more than monuments to wealth and charity: they were part of what he called a 'Police Architectonical', an architectural re-ordering which would embody and inculcate an awareness of the kind of urban environment which was necessary for civic health.[28]

Even so, there was an inevitable reaction against these baroque splendours and the 'vain magnificence of buildings'. Architectural extravagances seemed to one critic 'so many monuments of ill-gotten riches, attended with late repentance': he clearly had Guy's Hospital, funded from the proceeds of speculation in South Sea Company stock, in mind. Far from expressing ideals of charity and welfare, 'pride and vanity' in building could well be thought to divert attention from real social problems and the proper objects of benevolence.[29] Reactions of this kind paved the way for a new episode, which culminated in the voluntary hospitals of the eighteenth century.

THE VOLUNTARY EPISODE

The vigour of charitable enterprise in London in the 1690s and first decade of the eighteenth century depended to a considerable degree on voluntary associations, and especially on those religious societies of laymen which have recently been the object of much historical research. They had their roots in the 1670s, particularly in the West End, where Anglican clergy faced both social problems outside the limits of the old city and competition from Dissent and Popery. One of them was Anthony Horneck, preacher as it happens at the Savoy, and he may have been influenced by German pietism. Even if he was not, the Anglican revival of what was termed 'practical divinity' certainly had later links with pietism, through its most important creation, the Society for Promoting Christian Knowledge (SPCK), founded in 1699. Between 1706 and 1716 the Society published three influential tracts under the title *Pietas Hallensis* on the great pietist orphanage, hospital and school at Glaucha in Saxony.[30]

Voluntarism and practical divinity were not, of course, an

Anglican monopoly. Quakers and Dissenters with their own projects for employing and rehabilitating the poor might claim title to them. The two sides cooperated for a time, if only temporarily, in the Societies for Reformation of Manners which in the 1690s attacked moral and public nuisances – prostitution, profane swearing, trading on Sundays – again chiefly on the edges of the old city. But it was the SPCK, an exclusively Anglican Society, which in practice took the lead in sponsoring what came to be called 'associated philanthropy', the collection of regular subscriptions for new charitable purposes: first for charity schools, its greatest achievement; second for workhouses after 1715 when charity schools fell out of favour as potential nurseries of Jacobitism; and third for hospitals. Members of the SPCK were responsible for the foundation of the first of England's voluntary hospitals: the Westminster Hospital of 1720.[31]

The last thing the Society thought necessary, however, was another Chelsea, and a new hospital was far from being the initial intention. The founders of the Westminster, who included Henry Hoare, banker and stalwart of the SPCK, and High Churchmen like Samuel Wesley the younger, were members of the 'Charitable Society', originally set up in 1716 for 'the more easy and effectual relief of the sick and needy' by other means. Meeting weekly, their intention was to engage directly in the traditional works of mercy towards the 'poor wretch' who was 'a representative of Jesus Christ': to relieve poor strangers, visit prisoners, provide nurses for poor women in labour, and above all visit the sick and supply them with medicines and medical care. The provision of medicines was a fashionable charitable purpose, following the founding of two London dispensaries for the poor by the College of Physicians in 1696. But the Society's professed aims were religious rather than medical: 'to take care of the souls of those who are sick and needy, as well as of their bodies; it being certain that many poor people die without ever seeking, or receiving, the things which are necessary to their salvation'.[32]

This aspiration no doubt has a pietist ring to it, but it was also a theme which the Charitable Society shared with current philanthropy in Counter-Reformation France; and it may even have been borrowed from there. The first publication of the Charitable Society seems in fact to have very largely been based on a French tract which plainly belongs to the movement for *bureaux de charité* and general hospitals, supported by *Filles* and *Dames de la Charité*, which affected much of France from the 1680s.[33] The proposed 'sisters' of the Charitable Society who were to visit the sick were exactly like the *Dames de la Miséricorde* in Montpellier; and in 1726 the SPCK sponsored an English translation of a work on the hospitals and fraternities of Turin by the Jesuit Andrea Guevarre, who had been active in Montpellier and much of southern France.[34] In this case it was not Protestant Halle but Catholic towns of Southern Europe which provided explicit foreign models to be emulated.

Between 1716 and 1719, however, the Society turned its attention away from face-to-face charity by its members to the founding of an 'infirmary' for the 'sick and needy' of Westminster. It may be that brothers and sisters willing to visit the sick were less easy to find in London than in Montpellier or Turin. It certainly seems probable that well-to-do subscribers to a new institution were easier to recruit than volunteers for the dirty and perhaps dangerous work of door-to-door visiting. There was also another French, though this time Protestant, influence pushing in the same direction, in the shape of the Huguenot community in London, which was setting up the French Protestant Hospital, *La Providence*, chartered in 1718. At the same time, John Bellers, the Quaker pamphleteer and philanthropist, was turning from promoting workhouses to advocating the 'improvement of physic' by means of teaching hospitals, hospitals for incurables and for 'every capital distemper'.[35] The Westminster Hospital of 1720 was part of a general public interest in the medical contribution to metropolitan welfare, which Hartlib and his successors such as William Petty had long ago advocated, and of which they would have thoroughly approved.

This refocusing of philanthropy in a decisively medical direction, followed as it ultimately was by the founding of voluntary hospitals all over England, looks like the start of something new. In retrospect it was indeed the beginning, though only the remote beginning, of the modern hospital. In its early eighteenth century context, however, its links with the past are more obvious. Guy's Hospital, intended initially for incurables, was exactly the same in intent as its neighbour St Thomas's had been. The Charitable Society's view of the poor sick as 'representatives' of Christ was little different from Bishop Ridley's determination when supporting the civic hospitals in Edward VI's reign that 'Christ should lie no more abroad in the streets'.[36] More striking still was the Foundling Hospital, erected in London in 1739, but first planned by Thomas Coram in 1722, supported by Thomas Bray of the SPCK, and as indebted to French models as the Charitable Society. This was a straight replacement for the original Christ's Hospital which had been forced by the pressure of settlement legislation and the parochial relief system to refuse admission to foundlings in the later seventeenth century.[37]

In looking, as Thomas Guy did, for objects 'which the charity of others had not reached',[38] the founders of eighteenth-century hospitals were doing precisely the same thing as those rebuilding Bedlam for the insane in the 1670s, as Hartlib stressing the need to educate poor children when the London Corporation of the Poor was first discussed in the 1640s, and as the aldermen erecting five London hospitals for different purposes in the 1540s. They were rekindling traditional Christian charity, seeking new targets for it, and in doing so rediscovering the past.

The five episodes I have discussed, in necessarily truncated form, leave us with three general issues on which to reflect.

1 First and most obviously, and perhaps tritely, they show that new mechanisms for the protection of health and welfare had little to do with the social circumstances of poverty and disease themselves, and more to do with ideology and politics. So far as ideology is concerned, it was not so much a matter of secular as against religious ideals, or of Protestant as against Catholic varieties of Christianity: all could be turned in much the same directions. It was a matter of varying interpretations of Christian charity, and of different versions of the balance which always has to be struck in charitable activity: between, on the one hand, the disciplines necessary for the moral good of the recipient, and on the other, the sympathy and indulgence – the humility and benevolence – which Christian ethics dictate to be necessary for the good of the soul of the donor. As for politics, much obviously depended on power and the impetus to demonstrate it: on the relative influence and confidence at any moment of the central state (whether crown or parliament), civic government, parish authorities and the political parties which in the later part of the period influenced all of them.

2 Second, these various episodes have all exhibited London's place in a European intellectual environment. Foreign influences were often exerted close to home, by the French and Dutch refugee churches, but they did not need that intermediary. After an early phase, when Renaissance Italy provided the model, as it did elsewhere, governors and projectors looked directly to either Paris or the

Low Countries and Germany, and often to both. This ambivalence is predictable enough in early Stuart or Restoration England when kings naturally wanted a capital city like that of the Bourbons while some of their subjects wanted a Reformed citadel. It is more surprising to find the new Catholic philanthropy of the Counter-Reformation at least as influential as German pietism in Augustan and early Hanoverian London. It would be interesting to know whether trends in Southern Europe had an impact elsewhere in the Protestant north, and whether London contributed anything in repayment of its debts to continental cities.

3 Third and finally, it should be stressed that all of my episodes, from the 1550s onwards, were essentially superstructures, resting on the foundations of a parochial relief system which took care of most symptoms of social distress. To this extent they were a luxury in which London could afford to indulge, options which its rulers could discuss and debate without any profound sense of crisis. By 1696, poor rates in the City were raising something like £40,000 a year, and charitable benefactions, controlled by parishes and livery companies, probably producing an annual income of at least the same amount.[39] These sums, disbursed locally in face-to-face outdoor relief, help to explain parts of my story. With that kind of generous foundation to its welfare system, London had less need than other cities for charitable religious fraternities, or for effective centralisation – whether for the civic or the metropolitan entity, or for an effective combination of Bridewell and the Savoy such as a French *Hôpital-Général* might provide. Perhaps my episodes failed to do more than scratch the surface of real problems, because those problems were being managed – not completely successfully, but successfully enough – at the neighbourhood level, in other ways.

NOTES

1 Nicholas Hawksmoor, *Remarks on the Founding and Carrying on the Buildings of the Royal Hospital at Greenwich*, London 1728, 6.

2 This paper is published essentially in the form in which it was delivered. I hope to substantiate and develop some of the points in it, at greater length than is possible here, in a later publication.

3 Carole Rawcliffe, 'The Hospitals of Later Medieval London', *Medical History*, 28 (1984), 1–21; Jean Imray, *The Charity of Richard Whittington*, London 1968.

4 H. M. Colvin (ed.) *The History of the King's Works*, vol. III, 1485–1660 (Part I), London 1975, 196–201; Katharine Park and John

Henderson, ' "The First Hospital Among Christians": the Ospedale di Santa Maria Nuova in early sixteenth-century Florence', *Medical History*, 35 (1991), 164–88; John Henderson, 'The hospitals of Late-Medieval and Renaissance Florence: a preliminary survey', in Lindsay Granshaw and Roy Porter (eds) *The Hospital in History*, London 1989, 74–5.

5 *Memoranda, References and Documents relating to the Royal Hospitals of the City of London*, London 1836, Appendix, 1–4; Thomas Bowen, *Extracts from the Records and Court Books of Bridewell Hospital*, London 1798, Appendix, 1–2. On the refounding of the hospitals more generally, see Paul Slack, 'Social Policy and the Constraints of Government, 1547–1558', in Jennifer Loach and Robert Tittler (eds) *The Mid-Tudor Polity c. 1540–60*, London 1980, 108–13.

6 *Memoranda*, Appendix, 5; William Lempriere, *John Howes' MS, 1582*, London 1904, 9, 17.

7 *Memoranda*, Appendix, 57.

8 Bowen, *Extracts*, Appendix, 4. Cf. Joan Thirsk, *Economic Policy and Projects*, Oxford 1978, Chapter 2.

9 Pieter Spierenburg, *The Prison Experience: disciplinary institutions and their inmates in early modern Europe*, New Brunswick 1991, Chapter 3.

10 Paul Slack, *Poverty and Policy in Tudor and Stuart England*, London 1988, 121–2, 129.

11 R. H. Tawney and E. Power (eds) *Tudor Economic Documents*, London 1924, iii, 441–2; *Orders Appointed to be Executed in the Cittie of London, for Setting Rogues and Idle Persons to Work...*, London 1582, sig. Bi^v; Ian W. Archer, *The Pursuit of Stability: social relations in Elizabethan London*, Cambridge 1991, 238–43, 251–6.

12 *Orders appointed*, sig. Bii^v.

13 Valerie Pearl, 'Puritans and Poor Relief: the London workhouse, 1649–60', in Donald Pennington and Keith Thomas (eds) *Puritans and Revolutionaries: essays in seventeenth-century history presented to Christopher Hill*, Oxford 1978, 214–15; O. Grell, *Dutch Calvinists in Early Stuart London: the Dutch Church in Austin Friars 1603–42*, Leiden 1989, 47.

14 A. L. Beier and Roger Finlay (eds) *The Making of the Metropolis: London 1500–1700*, London 1986, 45, 48, 71; Slack, *Poverty and Policy*, 70.

15 Pearl, 'Puritans and Poor Relief', gives a full account of the Interregnum Corporation of the Poor.

16 Sheffield University Library, Hartlib papers, 15/2/35, 15/2/47. (The Hartlib papers are quoted from transcripts prepared by the Hartlib Papers Project, University of Sheffield, and quoted by permission of the Project Directors and the University Librarian.) On Corselis, see O. Grell, J. I. Israel and N.Tyacke (eds) *From Persecution to Toleration: the Glorious Revolution and religion in England*, Oxford 1991, 113.

17 Hartlib papers, 57/4/5A; Leonard Lee, *A Remonstrance Humbly presented to the High and Honourable Court of Parliament...*, London 1644, 12.

18 C. H. Firth and R. S. Rait (eds) *Acts and Ordinances of the Interregnum 1642–60*, London 1911 ii, 105; Pearl, 'Puritans and Poor Relief', 225–6.

19 House of Lords Record Office, Main Papers, 3 July 1661, 10 April 1662; *Journals of the House of Commons*, viii, 1660–7, 366; *Statutes of the Realm*, 13 and 14 Car. II, c. 12, sect. iv.

20 R. Latham and W. Matthews (eds) *The Diary of Samuel Pepys*, London 1970–83, v, 289; Stephen Macfarlane, 'Social Policy and the Poor in the Later Seventeenth Century', in Beier and Finlay, *Making of the Metropolis*, 258–63.

21 Craig Rose, 'Politics and the London Royal Hospitals, 1683–92', in Granshaw and Porter, *The Hospital in History*, 123–48; E. H. Pearce, *Annals of Christ's Hospital*, London 1901, 163–5; Craig Rose, 'Evangelical Philanthropy and Anglican Revival: the charity schools of Augustan London, 1698–1740', *London Journal*, 16 (1991), 35–65.

22 E. G. O'Donoghue, *The Story of Bethlehem Hospital*, London 1914, 210.

23 T. F. Reddaway, *The Rebuilding of London after the Great Fire*, London 1940, 249; W. G. Bell, *The Great Fire of London in 1666*, London 1920, 225, 277; O'Donoghue, *Bethlehem Hospital*, 192–5, 210–14; R. A. Aubin (ed.) *London in Flames, London in Glory*, New Brunswick 1943, 246.

24 *London in Flames*, 247; O'Donoghue, *Bethlehem Hospital*, frontispiece; M. I. Batten, 'The Architecture of Dr Robert Hooke FRS', *Walpole Society*, xxv (1937), 92.

25 Robert Somerville, *The Savoy. Manor: Hospital: Chapel*, London 1960, 72–3; returns to the 1665 survey in Lambeth Palace Library, MSS 639 and 951.

26 C. G. T. Dean, *The Royal Hospital Chelsea*, London 1950, 22–43; Christopher Clay, *Public Finance and Private Wealth: the career of Sir Stephen Fox, 1627–1716*, Oxford 1978, 133–8.

27 J. D. Thompson and G. Goldie, *The Hospital: a social and architectural history*, New Haven 1975, 84, 86, 147–9; John Woodward, *To Do the Sick no Harm: a study of the British voluntary hospital system to 1875*, London 1974, 14–15.

28 Hawksmoor, *Remarks*, 7.

29 *Proposals For Establishing a Charitable Fund in the City of London*, 2nd ed., London 1706, 21; Donna Andrew, *Philanthropy and Police: London charity in the eighteenth century*, Princeton NJ 1989, 26–7, note 42, and 33.

30 John Spurr, 'The Church, the Societies and the Moral Revolution of 1688', and Craig Rose, 'The Origins and Ideals of the SPCK 1699–1716', in John Walsh, Colin Haydon and Stephen Taylor (eds) *The Church of England c. 1689–c.1833*, Cambridge 1993, 127–42, 172–90; Augustus Hermann Francke, *An Abstract of the Marvellous Footsteps of Divine Providence... At Glaucha*, London 1706; *idem, Pietas Hallensis: Or, An Abstract...Part II*, London 1710; *idem, Pietas Hallensis...Part III*, London 1716.

31 R. B. Shoemaker, *Prosecution and Punishment: petty crime and the law in London and rural Middlesex c. 1660–1725*, Cambridge 1991, Chapter 9; M. G. Jones, *The Charity School Movement*, Cambridge 1938, Chapter II; Tim Hitchcock, 'Paupers and Preachers: the SPCK and the parochial workhouse movement', in Lee Davison *et al.* (eds) *Stilling the*

Grumbling Hive: the response to social and economic problems in England, 1689–1750, Stroud 1992, 145–66; Adrian Wilson, 'The Politics of Medical Improvement in Early Hanoverian London', in Andrew Cunningham and Roger French (eds) *The Medical Enlightenment of the Eighteenth Century*, Cambridge 1990, 10–24.

32 J. G. Humble and P. Hansell, *The Westminster Hospital 1716–1966*, London 1966, 11; *The Charitable Society: or, A Proposal For the More Easy and Effectual Relief of the Sick and Needy*, London 1715, sigs. A2–3, 13, 26; [?]Patrick Cockburn, *A Charitable Proposal For Relieving the Sick & Needy, And other Distressed Persons*, London 1719, 5–8; Albert Rosenberg, 'The London Dispensary for the Sick-Poor', *Journal of the History of Medicine*, 14 (1959), 41–56.

33 A manuscript note in the Bodleian Library, Oxford, copy of *The Charitable Society*, 1715, shelf-mark 24768 e.13, states that it is a translation of the 'substance' of 'a French sermon concerning infirmaries', though the note itself must be dated 1736 or later.

34 Colin Jones, *Charity and bienfaisance. The treatment of the poor in the Montpellier region 1740–1815*, Cambridge 1982, 49–50, 54; Andrea Guevarre, *Ways and Means For Suppressing Beggary And Relieving the Poor...*, London 1726.

35 A. G. Browning, 'On the Origin and Early History of the French Protestant Hospital (La Providence)', *Proceedings of the Huguenot Society of London*, vi (1898–1901), 43, 47, 53; George Clarke (ed.) *John Bellers: his life, times and writings*, London 1987, 179–82, 187.

36 *Tudor Economic Documents*, ii, 312.

37 Ruth K. McClure, *Coram's Children: the London Foundling Hospital in the eighteenth century*, New Haven CT 1981, 8–9, 19–22.

38 Woodward, *To Do the Sick no Harm*, 15.

39 Macfarlane, 'Social policy and the poor', 255, 257. Maitland's calculations of 1738 suggest that expenditure on the poor from metropolitan charitable endowments exceeded that from poor rates: William Maitland, *The History of London*, London 1739, 614, 634, 639, 682, 800.

Index